THE
HENRY HOLT
RETIREMENT
SOURCEBOOK

THE
HENRY HOLT
RETIREMENT
SOURCEBOOK

An Information Guide
for Planning and Managing
Your Affairs

WILBUR CROSS

A Henry Holt Reference Book

A STONESONG PRESS BOOK

HENRY HOLT AND COMPANY   NEW YORK

Library of Congress Cataloging-in-Publication Data
Cross, Wilbur.
The Henry Holt retirement sourcebook: an information guide for
planning and managing your affairs / by Wilbur Cross. — 1st ed.
p.   cm. — (A Henry Holt reference book)
"A Stonesong Press book."
Includes bibliographical references.
1. Retirement—United States—Planning.   I. Title   II. Series
HQ1063.2.U6C75 1991
646.7'9—dc20   91-17184
                                                        CIP
ISBN 0-8050-1760-7 (alk. paper)

Henry Holt Reference Books are available at special
discounts for bulk purchases for sales promotions, premiums,
fund-raising, or educational use. Special editions
or book excerpts can also be created to specification.
For details contact:
Special Sales Director, Henry Holt and Company, Inc.,
115 West 18th Street, New York, New York 10011.

First Edition—1992

Designed by Katy Riegel

Printed in the United States of America
Recognizing the importance of preserving
the written word, Henry Holt and Company, Inc.,
by policy, prints all of its first editions
on acid-free paper. ∞

1   3   5   7   9   10   8   6   4   2

CONTENTS

1

Introduction
to a Better Retirement

Whether the opportunities for retirement come earlier or later in your life, there are certain fundamentals that relate directly to the transition. As a lifestyle with choices that may not be familiar and with increased freedoms, retirement requires role modifications that are difficult for some people to make. So don't be hesitant about getting advice from other people who have retired and from organizations that are well qualified. These include private, nonprofit organizations; federal, state, and county agencies; clearinghouses of information; professionals who volunteer their services to older and retired people; and public and private libraries of many kinds.

This guidebook has been prepared to help you locate organizations that publish pertinent information on retirement and aging, provide referrals to other sources and resources, and in many cases offer specific assistance, sometimes at little or no cost. As many people who have retired are the first to admit, successful retirement is a matter of doing your homework and compiling as many facts as possible about what you want to do, how you want to spend your time, and where you want to be. You have to plan for this vital event in four ways: psychologically, by keeping in mind that retirement is not a passive state but one that is filled with fresh outlooks and expanded by new friends; physically, by being realistic about what your body can and cannot do; emotionally, by determining the best ways to love and receive love from relatives of all ages and by developing friends who are compatible and sympathetic; and financially, by setting aside enough to live on and by providing future income, and by choosing a retirement site that is appropriate to the kind of lifestyle you can really afford.

Planning your retirement is much like buying a home. You have to identify your needs and desires and lay out plans to accommodate them. Not only does retirement planning look ahead to the future—near or distant—it is also a remarkably effective way to engage in some self-analysis. As you consider retirement you can step back from the facts and frustrations of daily life, the demands of work and family that have set your priorities for so long. Now you can consider what is important to you. What do you really want out of life? With whom do you prefer to associate? What kind of environment would best suit the activities you wish to pursue? How can you ensure better health and emotional stability for yourself? Few people really know their goals and priorities well until they sit down and start evaluating them in terms of what they can accomplish in retirement.

When you feel confident that you have reviewed all the alternatives and covered all the bases, you almost automatically assure yourself of the best possible retirement. You retain your self-respect and build your image. Your attitude will become positive, and you will find that your relationships with other people become stronger and more meaningful. Hugh Downs, comparing his very successful and satisfying television career with the future he envisions for himself, wrote that "Retirement today is the beginning of a new, lengthy, important stage of life, rich with promise and well worth planning for."

If he can look forward to a new life with such obvious enthusiasm, then surely those of us whose careers may have been considerably less rewarding can expect retirement to be a marvelous change for the better.

Professional consultants working in the kinds of organizations you find in this resource book emphasize that there are six basic conditions that determine when, where, and how to retire:

• *Health.* People in good health say they want to retire while they can still enjoy life; those in failing health feel that a more leisurely lifestyle will be easier on them physically and may even reverse, or at least minimize, physical decline. In either case, health is the most important factor in a predominant number of cases in determining the quality of retirement.

• *Income.* Would-be retirees foresee that they will have an adequate retirement income. The ones who have plenty of money enjoy being able to pick and choose locations and housing at will. Those with limited income must be more selective and may well have to make a few sacrifices. Many retirees, however, are able to enjoy themselves even on limited budgets.

• *Spouse.* The husband, wife, or other partner is positively inclined toward retirement. When two people are involved, retirement works best when both are enthusiastic about assuming the new lifestyle and managing all aspects of it in a forthright and positive manner. Problems can develop if one partner looks upon retirement as fruitless, boring, or inferior to their former lifestyle.

• *Peer pressure.* Friends and associates in the same general age and social category are promoting retirement—and their particular style of retirement—as the right course of action. While the individuals concerned must, in the end, be the judges and make up their own minds, it is important to have a support group made up of relatives and friends alike who give the venture their blessing and, if need be, their assistance.

• *Psychological need.* Retirement suggests itself as the condition in life best suited to satisfying social needs and yearnings to pursue activities that are different from those of the past. Retirement for its own sake is not enough, and people making the decision whether or not to do so must realize that there are many individuals who could never be happy in retirement.

▪ *Family relationships.* Retirement promises closer ties with children and other relatives and more time in which to strengthen relationships that may have loosened over the years. This factor, though not usually the foremost one in reaching a decision, can be very meaningful. Many retirees have found to their pleasure— and sometimes to their surprise—that they finally got to know family members and other relatives in ways they never dreamed about before retiring.

If you have carefully considered these six factors before reaching the decision to retire, you are probably making a wise choice. However, before taking the final step, you do need to find reliable answers to any questions you have. This sourcebook provides as much practical and pertinent data as you can get. Refer to the capsule comments about the organizations and sources described later in this book. For most of these entries, you will find addresses and phone numbers. Phone numbers have been omitted, though, when organizations have requested that contacts be made only by mail, or in cases where such numbers change frequently. Please bear in mind, too, that some of the smaller organizations change their addresses periodically. This guidebook provides plenty of backup entries, so if you cannot find the answers you seek in one reference, try another.

As a starter, the following organizations can provide general information about aging and retirement:

American Association of Retired Persons

American Society on Aging

Council for the Elderly

Facts on File

Family Service America

Family Service Association

Gray Panthers

Mature Outlook

National Center on Arts and the Aging

National Council of Senior Citizens

National Council on the Aging

National Institute of Age, Work, and Retirement

National Institute of Senior Centers

National Institute on Aging

National Interfaith Coalition on Aging

Older Women's League

Social Security Administration

Veterans Administration

2

Location

According to the American Association of Retired Persons (AARP), almost 80 percent of the older people in the United States decide to stay put when they retire. However, many retirees would be better off if they moved and could thus adjust themselves better to changing needs. Yet they fail to make that choice, out of fear or inertia, or both. Some of the most commonplace reasons people choose not to move are: they cannot face the disruption of selling and moving; they are hesitant about trying to make new friends in an unfamiliar setting; they are afraid their children, other relatives, or some close friends will resent their move or be upset that they are leaving; they have heard horror stories about retirees who moved to supposed Shangri-La communities only to find out that the developer was going bankrupt or badly misrepresenting the housing and facilities; they have never made a major move in their entire lives and aren't even going to consider the idea.

Still, there are very good reasons for staying where you are. You may wish to remain near children and grandchildren. You may have established friendships and a place in your community that will satisfy you for a lifetime. And you may find the atmosphere, social and physical environments, and opportunities for growth are still just right for you in this new phase of your life.

Even if your present community seems perfect for your future, your present house might not be. What has been home for many years of your life, with children coming and going and perhaps one or more parents in residence for a time, may not always be suitable for retirement for a couple electing to remain in the same community. Yet there are plenty of options, which you can learn about in detail through organizations such as those listed in Chapter 3 of this resource book.

If, however, you decide that now is the time to move, how do you determine which location is right for you? There is only one way to do it properly and effectively, and that is to make a complete checklist of factors that are important to you and weigh them by how meaningful they are. For instance, Florida and southern California both offer warm climates, but the lifestyles are very different. You can have a rural life in either Vermont or Montana, but which climate do you prefer?

You must consider realistically all the variables that will determine how well you adapt to, and enjoy, your new life. These variables include the environment—where you can feel at home and where you can anticipate what will occur during an average day; the climate—where the surroundings are compatible with the activities you hope to pursue; and health benefits—such as a maximum of moderate-cost health-care facilities and a minimum of hazards and conditions that aggravate chronic ailments. Other considerations are the cost of living and your economic security; the prospects of what your personal image and identity will be among neighbors and newfound friends; the number and quality of sports and recreational programs that fit your needs; and the availability of services for older people.

Also consider: transportation and the accessibility of means to get from one place to another conveniently and inexpensively; cultural activities that will help you enlarge your horizons and make life more enjoyable; the availability of part-time jobs if you need to enhance your income; volunteer programs and other activities that can add new dimensions to your life now that you have more free time on your hands; courses and other educational opportunities; proximity to vacation areas that would be fun to visit on long weekends or holidays; and a reasonable amount of privacy and security.

How can you be certain of what you are getting into? How do you check out a community that *seems* to have the right environment, the facilities, and the advantages you are really seeking? Your first source of information is most likely to be relatives, friends, or friends of friends who already live there. In this case, you have to satisfy yourself about the reliability of their opinions. Can they be objective enough after having lived there to evaluate the pros and cons? Or are they lonely and homesick and hoping to lure friends there to try to enhance their own lives?

For specific data on locations, visit your local library and ask the reference librarian where you can find books on the state or community you have in mind. The listings of organizations in this resource book suggest publications of many kinds that will be informative in this respect, as does the the bibliography at the end of this book. The listings will also indicate private and public agencies, associations, and other organizations that can answer your questions directly by phone or mail, as well as through publications.

Even with these facts in hand, allow yourself time to reconnoiter at your leisure. You should plan exploratory trips to the region, spending less time at the recreation centers and more time checking out practical matters: markets, churches, the post office, the library, the Chamber of Commerce, the hospital, medical offices, and whatever types of organizations and services that have been most valuable to you in your present community. If you like the place but still are not totally sure that it is for you, try renting for a few months the kind of housing you have in mind for possible permanent residence. This is a safe and sane way to determine whether you are on target. The following is an initial list of the organizations in this book that can be helpful to you in selecting a retirement location:

Alliance to Save Energy

American Allergy Association

American Association of Retired Persons

American Automobile Association

American Financial Services Association

American Lung Association

American Mobilehome Association

Asthma and Allergy Foundation of America

Citizens for a Better Environment

Consumer Information Center

Council of Better Business Bureaus

Environmental Protection Agency

Federal Trade Commission

Gray Panthers

Mature Outlook

Money Management Institute

National Council of Senior Citizens

National Crime Prevention Council

National Moving and Storage Association

US Department of Housing and Urban Development

3

Your Choice of Residence

When you make a decision to retire, you are almost forced to ask yourself just what kind of residence would be most suited to your housing needs, your physical condition, and your pocketbook. You may consider your present residence a fine retirement home. Yet, before making the decision to remain where you are, take an inventory of the condition of the equipment and facilities in the house. How old is the plumbing? How obsolete the kitchen? How hazardous the electrical system? If you find a long list of things that need doing, you might be better off moving than trying to cope.

If you decide to remain in your present home but are concerned that it will be too expensive to maintain properly on a reduced budget, there are a number of options to consider, such as making part of the house into an apartment that can be rented on a long-term basis, renting one or two rooms to students or a young couple trying to survive in your community on a tight budget, closing off part of the house to reduce costs of heating and upkeep, establishing a small business that can be run from your home without conflicting with zoning laws, or considering a "reverse-mortgage" plan or home-equity loan to provide needed financing.

If you have decided to move to a new location, you will have a wealth of options to choose from. You can buy a single-family house, either as is or with repairs and improvements. The advantage is that you can know exactly what you are getting and determine how your present furniture will fit in. You might consider buying half of a two-family house owned by a younger couple willing to assume responsibility for exterior maintenance for a modest fee, thus cutting the initial cost and phasing out the yardwork. You can build a new home designed to your specifications on property that is in a location of your choice, but you must keep close tabs on mounting costs not in the original estimate. You should also consider a town house or villa, the type that is conventionally joined with one or more similar units, and which involves less maintenance outside. Or you could picture yourself in a condominium where there is almost no exterior work at all.

Many retirees have been happy with a retirement community, where everything is made to order for people who want to minimize household chores and repair problems. These differ widely by type and cost but are similar in that they are designed to offer older people the best housing, services, social life, and facilities with the least amount of work commitment and risk. Residents, however, have to be willing to surrender a certain degree of privacy and independence and must feel comfortable with group activities.

A new approach to the housing dilemma for retired people is homesharing, a concept that was in its infancy at the beginning of the 1980s but has been increasing steadily in popularity. Homesharing is an arrangement whereby one residence is shared by two or more individuals, couples, or families. There are numerous patterns of ownership and responsibilities for sharing the economic burden, such as taxes, mortgages, maintenance, and repairs. Homesharing—shared housing—is particularly appropriate for retired people who are single and want to assure a degree of companionship while maintaining their privacy and keeping living costs in line.

Whichever housing arrangement seems the most attractive, money usually influences the decision the most. Consultants in listed organizations dealing with housing recommend that you ask yourselves these questions: What percent of your income have you been spending on housing recently? Is the amount you have been spending minimal, adequate, or quite comfortable? What is your anticipated annual budget for housing during the next five years? Do you expect your income to increase or decrease during that five-year period? Would an arrangement that brought in rental income from an accessory apartment be worth the modification cost or change in lifestyle? Would the financial benefits of living with others be worth adapting to a new kind of living arrangement? What would happen if you should need special health care?

When you make your decision about a retirement home, bear in mind that certain features may be unsuitable, or even unsafe, for older people. Retirees generally prefer all rooms on the same level, with a minimum of stairs, thresholds, or other traffic hazards; bathrooms located close to and in a direct route from bedrooms, not only for quick, easy access but to avoid any stumbling and fumbling in the dark; safety-type bathroom fixtures and grips; floors with nonslip surfaces and an absence of loose scatter rugs; improved lighting and easy-to-find switches; halls at least forty-eight inches wide and doorways thirty inches wide to accommodate wheelchairs, if necessary; easy-opening doors with locks that cannot be set accidentally; storage areas and closets that are easy to reach and shelves no higher than six feet above the floor level, to prevent having to stretch; acoustical controls to muffle exterior noises and prevent interior sounds that interfere with speech and hearing; comfortable heating and air-conditioning; ventilation that filters out pollens, air pollutants, and odors; exterior steps with sturdy, grippable handrails, well-marked edges, and proper lighting; and garages that have remote-control automatic doors, proper lighting, good ventilation, and storage areas that help to avoid clutter.

Many of the organizations in the listings can provide basic data and good suggestions for retirement housing. The following are good places to start:

Alliance to Save Energy

American Mobilehome Association

Citizens for a Better Environment

Consumer Information Center

Environmental Protection Agency

Family Service America

Family Service Association

Household International

Money Management Institute

National Association for Home Care

National Crime Prevention Council

National Fire Protection Association

National Foundation for Consumer Credit

National Moving and Storage Association

National RV Owners Club

National Shared Housing Resource Center

US Department of Housing and Urban Development

4

Toward
a More Healthful
Retirement

Good health and retirement can go hand in hand for those who
do their homework and plan their lives realistically. In spite of the
dismal picture many people have of being "elderly," statistics
show that eight out of ten Americans sixty-five or older are in
excellent, good, or fair health. And only 5 percent of these seniors
live in nursing homes or similar institutions. It is promising to
learn that the majority of retired people are well and living perfectly normal—if not better than normal—lives.

The only negative statistic is that health care can become a
costlier item in the budget after the age of sixty-five. Yet you can
still take positive steps to maintain good health, keep costs in line,
and pursue fitness programs that are effective. Organizations in
the medical/health field report that most of today's health problems result from unfortunate lifestyle choices rather than from
aging, citing poor nutrition, smoking, lack of exercise, reactions to
stress, and the misuse of drugs and alcohol as the real culprits.
Many of the problems commonly attributed to growing old can
be minimized, halted, even reversed through changes in lifestyle.
What better time to take a positive step than when retiring!

Aging is not always a declining process, even though it may require people to slow down and relax. A great deal depends upon your outlook and the way you act, rather than on your score on a physical test. If you are like other older people who are retired, or are planning to retire, you consider the state of your health as one of the major considerations in deciding where to retire. Even more important than where you live is *how* you live. Organizations devoted to the welfare of older people advise their members to *stay active*. Boredom is the retiree's greatest enemy. Those who avoid its clutches are the ones who develop hobbies and other interests and become involved in activities that keep their minds and bodies active, and thus help maintain sound mental and physical health at any age.

The Aging Health Policy Center at the University of California offers an important clue to the relationship between health and retirement. Aging, it reports, is often defined as a decreased ability to adapt to the environment. This definition is quite different from the chronological one because it recognizes the important differences in physical capacity at different ages and among persons of the same age.

One of the first things people do when they get ready to retire is worry about health problems and illness. It is only natural to consider what the effects of aging will be on your health, since seniors do suffer from some conditions more than they did when they were younger. In order of prevalence, the illnesses that most affect people when they reach retirement age are: arthritis, hypertension, heart condition, sinus disorders, orthopedic problems, vision impairment, and diabetes. Yet research data show that only about one out of ten older Americans is significantly disabled by chronic health conditions. And many seniors who are so afflicted manage to cope perfectly well, often suffering only minor aches and pains, or annoyances, as they follow the advice of their doctors.

Another common concern for older people is the cost of staying healthy or countering a specific disease. While it is true that health costs generally increase for senior citizens, there are steps you can take to help maintain a reasonable budget. Among the steps advocated by health groups that counsel retirees are these: Select doctors who accept Medicare assignments and are sympathetic to the financial problems of older people; renew prescriptions only as needed, and discontinue them as soon as possible; buy generic drugs; never undergo surgery without getting a second opinion; check your health and medical policies to make sure you are not paying for double coverage; apply for all benefits to which you are entitled, and appeal any substantial rejection of Medicare or medical insurance for a specific service. Above all, study and practice every feasible way you can to take better care of your health through preventive measures, such as active exercise and a healthful diet.

The following organizations, among many others listed in this book, can be helpful in supplying you with information, advice, and appropriate reading on medicine and health in retirement.

American Allergy Association

American Association of Foot Specialists

American Cancer Society

American Council of Life Insurance

American Dental Association

American Health Care Association

American Heart Association

American Hiking Society

American Lung Association

American Medical Association

American Natural Hygiene Society

Arthritis Foundation

Asthma and Allergy Foundation of America

Better Hearing Institute

Better Vision Institute

Center for Consumer Health Education

Comprehensive Pain Center

Council on Family Health

Diet Workshop

Elder Health Program

Food Safety and Inspection Service

Footwear Council

Headache Research Foundation

Health Care Financing Administration

Heart Life

High Blood Pressure Information Center

Information for the Partially Sighted

Medic Alert

Mended Hearts

National Association for the Deaf

National Clearinghouse for Alcohol and Drug Abuse
    Information

National Diabetes Information Clearinghouse

National Eye Care Project

National Hospice Organization

National Institute of Dental Research

National Institute of Mental Health

National Institute on Aging

National Institutes of Health

National League for Nursing

National Mental Health Association

National Society to Prevent Blindness

Oral Health Research Center

Rehabilitation International

Self-Help for Hard-of-Hearing People

Society for Nutrition Education

US Department of Health and Human Services

US Food and Drug Administration

Vision Foundation

Vitamin Information Bureau

Walking Association

5

Physical Fitness and Sports

Think about all those times in the past when you've said to yourself, "I've got to lose a little of the flab. Take an exercise program. Get fit." And then added, "But I've got so many things to do—my job, the kids, the yardwork. I'll start my fitness program when I have a little more time and energy." Well, in retirement you actually have the time, as well as the motivation. And there's no better moment to start.

Exercise programs offer a multitude of health benefits. They neutralize whatever physical declines may be in progress, strengthen your heart, and upgrade your lung capacity. They also aid in relieving anxiety, improving mental alertness, helping you to sleep more soundly, and creating a sense of well-being. When planning for retirement, take stock of your personal health and establish a realistic fitness program. You don't have to jog two miles a day or lift weights or take up cross-country skiing. In fact, you should avoid action that is too strenuous and calls upon muscles and functions that have never been exerted before. The best exercises for older people are those that are rhythmic, vigorous, and continuous. Some examples are walking briskly, bicycling, swimming, skipping rope, and aerobic dancing.

Continuity and frequency are vital. You should exercise at least every other day and for periods of twenty to thirty minutes. Plan a program that is gradual and progressive: Avoid sudden start-ups and stops; include warm-up and cool-down periods of five to ten minutes, the length depending upon the duration and intensity of the exercises themselves. Good ways to warm up and finish are stretching, jogging in place, and light calisthenics.

Exercise programs can be as different as night and day, accomplishing a variety of health objectives. For instance, calisthenics and isometrics (strengthening muscles by pitting one against another) are great for improving muscle tone, strength, and flexibility, but will not improve lung and heart capacity. Aerobic exercises, on the other hand—ones that are rhythmic and continuous—stimulate the heart, tone the blood vessels, and build the lungs.

Many people who play popular sports, such as tennis, golf, and bowling, feel that they get enough exercise and thus do not have to schedule a fitness program. Those particular sports are fine, but they do not provide the benefits of aerobic exercises because they involve start-and-stop, rather than continuous, motion.

No matter how healthy you think you are, your plan must include an initial visit to your doctor, with whom you can discuss your retirement plans and your fitness goals. The American Medical Association recommends that all adults over fifty have a complete physical examination before they undertake any kind of exercise program. It is more vital than ever if you have not engaged in active sports recently, are overweight, experience back or joint discomfort, have hypertension, or have a history of heart disease or other serious illness. However, the fact that you have medical problems should not be an excuse to lapse into inactivity.

When you start a fitness program, do not just plunge in, but begin gradually and progressively; avoid straining your body; and get plenty of rest between exercises. It should take you about three months to phase into a full-scale program geared to your condition and capabilities. It is important to participate frequently, but even more so to be consistent and to precede each session with a warm-up and end with a cooling-down period. Be vigorous—you can exercise briskly without straining or risking muscle pulls.

You will see signs that you are making progress as you work yourself into suitable exercise programs, but don't expect immediate results. It takes time, particularly for older people who are trying to become fit after a sedentary life.

Many retired people report that the best exercise for them is walking, recommended by many doctors as a fine, safe way to keep the body in tone. Make walking a priority in your retirement program. The longer and more briskly you walk in a natural way and without feeling winded or pushed, the better off you will be. Many people find that the early hours are the best time for exercise because it is not interrupted by phone calls, daily chores, and other distractions. It is also one of the loveliest and most inspiring times, especially if you have moved to a retirement community that is in natural surroundings.

As you plan a retirement exercise program, you should also give serious thought to diet and nutrition. It is important to keep in mind that too much leisure time—which many retirees have—is likely to cause boredom and an urge to wander into the kitchen and nibble. Yet retirement also offers a natural opportunity to get better food, prepare it more carefully, and enjoy it more than ever before. You no longer have to rush meals and can spend more time purchasing and preparing foods that are both appetizing and healthful. Furthermore, many retirement areas have easy access to fresh fish or continuing harvests of healthful fruits and vegetables. Liquids are also essential, assisting greatly in the processes of digestion and regular elimination, as well as supplying needed nutrients. Health professionals suggest that older people drink at least two quarts a day, whether water, dairy drinks, fruit juices, or other liquids. That amounts to six to eight glasses, an amount that many people unfortunately take several days to consume.

For better health and fitness, the following is just a selective list of organizations from this book's master list that can provide detailed information, advice, and reading matter to help you reach your goals.

American Allergy Association

American Association of Foot Specialists

American Cancer Society

American Council of Life Insurance

American Dental Association

American Health Care Association

American Heart Association

American Hiking Society

American Lung Association

American Medical Association

American Natural Hygiene Society

Arthritis Foundation

Asthma and Allergy Foundation of America

Better Hearing Institute

Better Vision Institute

Center for Consumer Health Education

Comprehensive Pain Center

Council on Family Health

Diet Workshop

Elder Health Program

Food Safety and Inspection Service

Footwear Council

Headache Research Foundation

Health Care Financing Administration

Heart Life

High Blood Pressure Information Center

Information for the Partially Sighted

Life Care Society of America

Lifeline Systems

Medic Alert

Mended Hearts

National Association for the Deaf

National Clearinghouse for Alcohol and Drug Abuse Information

National Diabetes Information Clearinghouse

National Eye Care Project

National Hospice Organization

National Institute of Dental Research

National Institute of Mental Health

National Institute on Aging

National Institutes of Health

National League for Nursing

National Mental Health Association

National Society to Prevent Blindness

Oral Health Research Center

Rehabilitation International

Self-Help for Hard-of-Hearing People

Society for Nutrition Education

US Department of Health and Human Services

US Food and Drug Administration

Vision Foundation

Vitamin Information Bureau

Walking Association

6

Your Nutrition Program

Health organizations cite four basic food sources that provide a good balance for older people: proteins, such as meat, poultry, eggs, and fish; vegetables and fruits; dairy products, including milk products and cheeses; and breads and pastas. Retirees are advised generally not to follow food fads that specify an overconsumption of one or two of these basic sources, but to retain an overall balance.

Keep in mind, too, the following goals when planning meals and making food purchases: Vary your menu, rather than sticking to the same old foods day in and day out; choose the kinds of foods that help you maintain a constant weight; do some homework to find out which foods should be avoided because of saturated fat and cholesterol; limit intake of salt or sodium (try flavoring foods with lemon and herbs rather than salt and pepper); and add to the menu plenty of foods that are good sources of fiber and that provide adequate amounts of starch.

More and more food manufacturers, whether by edict or choice, are listing the makeup of their products in terms of sodium content, calories per serving, flavorings, and other ingredients. If you learn exactly what you are putting into your stomach, or what you are avoiding, you will be much better off in the long run. Many supermarkets now make it a practice to have sections with foods that are low in salt or that are particularly beneficial for dieters.

Only recently have older people come to know more about the value of fiber in their diets. Each year, nearly 100,000 Americans are diagnosed as having cancer of the colon. In addition to reducing the risk of colon cancer, increased fiber may also help to avoid diverticulitis and other bowel disorders and serve to relieve constipation.

In the matter of nutrition, older people should also check with their doctor to determine whether medications they are taking might change their dietary needs. The process of aging is such that the older body may not react well to certain combinations of foods and drugs. Even such seemingly beneficial actions as taking vitamins and minerals can cause unwanted interactions. Drugs can also affect your appetite, in severe cases causing nutritional difficulties. Also, some combinations of foods and drugs have adverse effects on your system—consuming milk, for example, within an hour or two of taking tetracycline, which reduces its potency, or drinking juice after taking penicillin, whose effectiveness is lessened by acids.

When it comes to diet, nutrition, and related health matters, the following organizations, among others, can be helpful in providing information and guidelines.

American Allergy Association

American Cancer Society

American Dental Association

American Health Care Association

American Heart Association

American Medical Association

American Natural Hygiene Society

Arthritis Foundation

Asthma and Allergy Foundation of America

Center for Consumer Health Education

Council on Family Health

Diet Workshop

Elder Health Program

Food Safety and Inspection Service

Heart Life

High Blood Pressure Information Center

National Clearinghouse for Alcohol and Drug Abuse
Information

National Diabetes Information Clearinghouse

National Institute of Dental Research

National Institute on Aging

National Institutes of Health

Oral Health Research Center

Society for Nutrition Education

Vitamin Information Bureau

US Department of Health and Human Services

US Food and Drug Administration

7

The Economics of Retirement

Although personal health tops the list of concerns for people who have retired or are about to, the subject of money runs a close second. Strangely, financial matters are often the first ones that are put off until "tomorrow" as too tough to cope with now. Many people feel that they are out of their depth when it comes to any aspect of economics. Besides, they just cannot face what they might see on that "bottom line" when they have totaled their assets and debits. Yet procrastination is perhaps the greatest single stumbling block on the way to a worry-free retirement.

Financial planning is essentially quite simple. You need a road map to show where you are, where you want to go, what your best route is for getting there, and how long it will take.

Many older people retire with the idea that they are never again going to have to face a job. Yet within a year of retiring they go back to work, either to generate income they find they need or to escape boredom and engage in more stimulating activity than they were able to find. Some try new and unfamiliar types of work because such jobs are available in the location to which they have retired. Others establish themselves as consultants in fields in which they have had experience and training. Is it all worth it? If you don't seriously need the income, you should consider whether you are perhaps sacrificing the very leisure you worked so hard and long to achieve.

When you retire, you relinquish a certain amount of financial control. You may no longer find it easy to switch to a new job or field of work or move freely from one kind of community or residence to another that is more suited to your budget. More and more, you may see financial matters slipping out of hand, and you begin asking yourself what you can and cannot do to stay on an even financial keel. One positive step is to determine which assets you can control, such as investments, and which are fixed and beyond changing, such as a pension. You also have to evaluate your debts and living expenses to determine how controllable each one of these may be. Ask yourself questions like these:

Are my (our) income-producing assets, such as securities, earning as much as they could? Should I switch from one kind of investment to another to reduce income taxes? Are any assets earning little, such as cash sitting in a checking account with little or no interest? Can living expenses be reduced without seriously upsetting my retirement lifestyle? Can any monthly debt payments be reduced substantially, perhaps by selling an asset that carries a large debt? Can income taxes and other taxes be reduced by keeping better records of deductible items?

If you have hangups about financial matters and find them difficult to discuss, let alone deal with, it might be worth your while to do some homework and seek professional guidance. The following organizations are examples from the master list of those that can provide information, reading matter, and further resources on financial matters and household budgets.

Active Corps of Executives (ACE)

AFL-CIO Community Services Department

American Association of Retired Persons Worker Equity
Department

American Bankers Association

American Council of Life Insurance

American Financial Services Association

Bankcard Holders of America

Consumer Information Center

Consumer Product Safety Commission

Consumers Union of the United States

Council of Better Business Bureaus

Credit Union National Association

Federal Deposit Insurance Corporation

Federal Trade Commission

Household International

Insurance Information Institute

Money Management Institute

National Association of Investors Corporation

National Consumers League

National Foundation for Consumer Credit

National Institute of Age, Work, and Retirement

National Self-Help Clearinghouse

Pension Rights Center

Service Corps of Retired Executives (SCORE)

Small Business Administration

United Seniors Health Cooperative

US Department of Labor

US Equal Employment Opportunity Commission

US Securities and Exchange Commission (SEC)

8

Your Legal Needs

When you retire, you naturally hope and expect that you will not require much help in the matter of legal issues and actions. However, there are many common matters that require some form of legal documentation, such as making a will; buying property; assigning power of attorney to a friend or relative to handle personal matters should you become incapacitated; establishing a business partnership; obtaining consumer credit to which you think you are entitled, particularly when moving to a new community; protesting questionable practices on the part of a firm that has sold you property in a retirement development; placing your property in joint ownership; and establishing a trust fund.

If you have moved to a new community, you may find that choosing the right lawyer is like trying to locate the right dentist or physician. You want someone who is compatible, proficient, readily available, yet reasonable when it comes to billing you for services rendered. In reverse order, your first step should most likely relate to costs. In some cases, you can use a paralegal (legal assistant) to undertake the bulk of the work at a lower rate than that charged by a practicing attorney. At the very least, ask about hourly rates and the estimated time required for the work to be done. This is perfectly proper, and you should avoid hiring any attorney who gives you evasive answers. You should enter any such discussion armed with a list and description of your specific needs. If they are complex and tricky, you might do better to select a lawyer whose hourly fee is on the high side but who is familiar with the subjects at hand and can complete his or her end of the bargain far more quickly than another lawyer whose rates are lower.

If you have several legal needs, you do not necessarily have to use the same lawyer for all of them. Bear in mind, too, that if you anticipate having a continuing number of legal problems, you might subscribe to one of a number of prepaid legal plans. These can be located through some of the organizations listed in this book, through a local bar association, or sometimes by looking in the state and county sections of the telephone directory for government offices listed under "Law" or "Legal." For as little as fifteen or twenty dollars a month, you can have almost unlimited consultations with lawyers who are members of the plan. This kind of service might be practical if you are planning to start your own business, buying a retail establishment, or serving as a consultant in a field in which you have to draw up proposals or recommend ways to expedite joint ventures.

The question frequently arises: When can I act as my own lawyer? In some routine cases, such as handling sales contracts or defining property rights-of-way with a neighbor, you can "be your own lawyer" in that you can do the necessary homework, draw up the documents required, and then have a legal clinic review your language to ascertain that it conforms to legal standards. The charge will be nominal and the clinic will make itself available to assist you should there be errors in your presentation. You can also, with the help of printed guides, draft a will and prepare other papers that are more or less standard. These might include taking a complaint to small claims court to obtain recompense for defective goods, asking for an official hearing if Medicare refuses to honor a claim, for example. In each case, though, you should make sure that you prepare thoroughly and carefully.

Also, do your homework. One way to start is to visit a law library and do a little research. Another is to get in touch with public and private nonprofit organizations that can assist you. A selection of these is listed below, excerpted from this book's master list.

Citizens Emergency Center

Commission on Civil Rights

Commission on Legal Problems of the Elderly

Community Action for Legal Services

Council of Better Business Bureaus

Legal Services for the Elderly

Major Appliance Consumer Action Panel

National Council Against Health Fraud

National Resource Center for Consumers of Legal
   Services

National Senior Citizens Law Center

Older Women's League

US Equal Employment Opportunity Commission

Volunteer Lawyers Project

9

Hobbies and Socio/Cultural Affairs

People look forward to retirement as a time when they are really going to be able to fulfill their desires, pursue hobbies, attend concerts, take up watercolor painting, build ship models, collect stamps, read great books, handcraft furniture, or grow prize-winning flowers in their gardens. Yet what often happens is that they sit around watching television, shuffle off to occasional sporting events, or drip away the time doing nothing much they can remember the next day.

With a little planning, though, retirement time—what we refer to as "leisure time"—can be fruitful, enjoyable, and even remunerative. The rewards are many, when you have planned in a positive way. The first step is finding out where the action is for you, and then getting involved. Experts all agree that the more active you are, the fewer problems you will have. Growing old is not the same as aging. There are far too many people in their fifties and even forties who are "aging" because they have nothing stimulating and constructive to do. So, go where the action is and you won't have to worry about being "too old." It is surprising to find out how many successful businesspeople in their seventies did not even start their ventures until they retired.

Many retirees have reaped their rewards from hobbies or latent talents they had in various cultural fields, such as art, music, or theater. Others delight in becoming entrepreneurs, starting a small business that may or may not be connected with a field in which they had previous experience. Although retirement advisors caution older people about taking on full-time work loads, the retirees who are successful often find the work just as relaxing as pursuing a hobby. If you find work to be both challenging and enjoyable, why forgo the pleasure and stimulation that it brings? You can always continue at a slower pace, working shorter hours and planning interim holiday and vacation periods.

A word of caution about hobbies is in order. An informal survey of retired men and women revealed the fact that the amount of money they spent on expensive equipment and supplies was inversely related to the enjoyment they seemed to derive from the hobby. Those with very expensive cameras, for example, worried too much about technical details, damaging their equipment, or having to insure everything against theft and loss. People who invested heavily in top-quality oil paints, fancy easels, and a needless array of brushes never quite seemed to get down to the business of painting. And those who tried to grow the most exotic flowers and plants instead of more common species were endlessly discouraged at the results of their labors.

The moral of all this is that you should start small even though you might want to think big. Then, if one hobby or pursuit proves to be disappointing or beyond your skills, you need not feel locked into it and unable to change horses in midstream. If you don't know where to start, try adult education programs as a means of learning things quickly.

For information about activities that can add dimension and stimulation to your retirement years, the following organizations might provide some initial information and guidance.

ACTION

American Craft Council

Association for Continuing Higher Education

Clearinghouse on the Handicapped

Elderhostel

Foster Grandparent Program

Garden Club of America

Grandparents Association of America

Institute of Lifetime Learning

National Amputee Golf Association

National Center on Arts and the Aging

National Fitness Foundation

National Self-Help Clearinghouse

National Senior Sports Association

President's Council on Physical Fitness and Sports

Service Corps of Retired Executives (SCORE)

Small Business Administration

Volunteer Talent Bank of the AARP

Volunteer: The National Center

10

Volunteerism and Community Activities

Regardless of their involvement with hobbies, cultural affairs, or even part-time jobs, more and more retired people are finding an ever stimulating and always rewarding way to spend their time: as volunteers. Keeping active in volunteer programs was described by one magazine for older readers as "a sure cure for the blues." According to a survey of subscription holders, this area of activity is considered by seniors to be the best way to prevent mental aging and to boost the spirits, energy, and outlook of people who get involved.

Retirement professionals support this viewpoint. One study revealed that when a group of volunteers was compared with a nonvolunteer group, the members of the former were, age for age, healthier mentally and physically and far more contented with their lot than those in the latter group. Furthermore, they felt far more secure emotionally because they tended to make new friends easily while volunteering. Those who worked in hospitals and other medical and health facilities enjoyed the added advantage of feeling that they were much more familiar with such resources should they themselves ever need help.

Opportunities for volunteer work are limitless, as well as very flexible. Participants can determine whether they want to be involved for just a few hours each week or almost daily. What you volunteer for depends in large part upon the work you feel will be most satisfying and productive, and how it relates to your personal interests, experience, skills, capabilities, and preferences. Among the most common organizations and institutions that solicit volunteers are hospitals, which match applicants' skills with local needs; libraries, which seldom have large enough budgets for many salaried employees; environmental agencies, which require regular help with recycling programs; Meals-on-Wheels and other shut-in programs that need help with preparation and transportation; nursing homes, which welcome anyone who can entertain patients, read to the visually impaired, or simply provide company; consumer-aid groups interested in spotting and taking action against frauds; public schools, which usually staff adult-education programs with volunteers; churches of every denomination; and senior-citizen centers, which are themselves almost totally staffed by volunteers.

Volunteers are increasingly essential to a broad range of social and community programs that would literally fold up without them. Programs to assist children from disadvantaged families, to help low-income, home-bound adults who are ill, and to provide transportation for the physically handicapped would be almost impossible without volunteers.

There are many sources of information for retired men and women who want to get involved. The following are but a few.

ACTION

American Craft Council

Association for Continuing Higher Education

Clearinghouse on the Handicapped

Elderhostel

Foster Grandparent Program

Garden Club of America

Grandparents Association of America

Institute of Lifetime Learning

National Center on Arts and the Aging

National Fitness Foundation

National Hospice Organization

National Institutes of Health

National Self-Help Clearinghouse

National Senior Sports Association

Service Corps of Retired Executives (SCORE)

Small Business Administration

Volunteer Talent Bank of the AARP

Volunteer: The National Center

YMCA and YWCA

11

Travel and Recreation

Just because you are retired does not mean that you don't need occasional vacations. Experts say that it is good for your health to get a change of environment and routine, even though you may be living in a community where other people deliberately come for holidays and recreation. Consider the advantages that retired people have over those who are still holding full-time jobs: they can travel during off-peak days and hours, thus avoiding crowds; they can more easily take advantage of discount periods; they can extend their stay without having to phone the boss if they find the vacation spot particularly attractive; they can participate in home-exchange plans if their own home is in a locale that vacationers from abroad would like to visit; and they are far more flexible in every respect when it comes to making or changing travel plans.

No matter how attractive their retirement location, most retirees benefit from vacations away from home. Many, of course, travel in order to visit children, grandchildren, and other relatives and friends, and that in itself can be fulfilling. Unless travel is physically difficult, you should have periodic holidays, if not full-fledged vacations, in your retirement calendar. Even if you have disabilities, however, do not discount the potential values of vacation travel. Increasing numbers of airlines, other carriers, hotels, and resorts provide special facilities for people who have physical or mental disorders, usually at no extra cost and sometimes at reduced rates. Many of the resources described in this book concern plans and accommodations of this kind.

Another benefit that comes from being retired and thinking about a trip is that you have the time to spend on doing your homework and making plans. In fact, well-traveled retirees report that the planning is half the fun of the trip itself. During this period, you can widen your horizons in a marvelous way. You can be as selective as you like, often gaining new and interesting insights into places and people to be encountered en route. Some retirees go so far as to sign up for adult-education programs on specific countries or to take language lessons if they are planning to go abroad. Others hold small dinner parties for friends and neighbors who have traveled in the regions selected and can provide useful information and tips about the land and the people.

If you are fortunate enough that money is no object, the world is your oyster. But don't be discouraged if your budget is tight. You can find many bargains in the travel field if you have the time, patience, and inclination to seek them out. As for domestic travel, most of the fifty states go all out on occasion to provide a taste of their attractions to older visitors. One typical example is Tennessee, which hosts an annual travel promotion known as "Senior Class" in September, during which more than five hundred restaurants, hotels, merchants, and sightseeing firms offer discounts and plan special events for older visitors. Williamsburg, Virginia, is another solicitor of older tourists. This restored colonial town sponsors "Senior Time" each year, and mails brochures to more than thirty thousand people who request them. And the federal government now makes "Golden Age Passports" available to all Americans over sixty-two for free entry to national parks and recreation areas.

No matter where or when you go, it pays to belong to a national organization like AARP, AAA, or Mature Outlook, whose members are from the older generation and are thus eligible for special travel and vacation packages, which combine extra benefits with discounted rates.

To discover the many advantages of retirement-oriented trips and vacations, consult the resources listed in this book. The following are good for starters.

American Association of Retired Persons (AARP)

American Automobile Association

American Bed and Breakfast Association

American Hiking Society

Boat Owners Association of the United States

Elderhostel

Healthcare Abroad

International Association for Medical Assistance to Travelers

Mature Outlook

National Amputee Golf Association

National Fitness Foundation

National RV Owners Club

National Senior Sports Association

President's Council on Physical Fitness and Sports

Public Health Service

Society for Advancement of Travel for the Handicapped

United States Tour Operators Association

Vacation and Senior Citizens Association

Walking Association

RETIREMENT
SOURCES

AAA Foundation   **AAAFTS**
for Traffic Safety
12600 Fair Lakes Circle
Fairfax, VA 22033

(703) 222-4104
(800) 763-6600

Profile: The AAA Foundation for Traffic Safety conducts studies on highway and traffic safety, makes reports, and encourages legislation to improve traffic safety. AAA members and others can benefit from foundation reports, as well as make inquiries.

Publications: The AAAFTS distributes reports and fact sheets based on its studies and on professional recommendations for highway and traffic safety.

ACTION
National Center for
Service Learning
1100 Vermont Avenue, NW
Washington, DC 20525

(202) 634-9380
(800) 424-8867

Profile: ACTION administers and coordinates domestic volunteer programs sponsored by the federal government. ACTION volunteers work throughout the country in programs that help meet basic needs and support self-help efforts of low-income individuals and communities. Many older people become involved through such ACTION-related groups as the Foster Grandparent Program (FGP), the Senior Companion Program (SCP), and the Retired Senior Volunteer Program (RSVP).

Publications: While there are no regular periodicals, communications are well maintained through newsletters, releases, and other occasional publications.

Action for Independent Maturity   **AIM**
1909 K Street, NW
Washington, DC 20049

(202) 872-4850

Profile: The goal of AIM is to provide useful information to people between the ages of fifty and sixty-five who are still actively employed but may be planning retirement in a few years.

Publications: AIM publications cover a multitude of subjects, including retirement, financial management, medicine and health, and the uses of leisure time.

Action for Older Persons   AOP
144 Washington Street
Binghamton, NY 13901

(607) 722-1251

Profile: Action for Older Persons is a nonprofit advocacy agency for seniors. It developed its Pre-Retirement Education Program (PREP) in 1974 to foster the exchange of useful information and ideas among participants. Programs and discussions cover the following topics, among others: opportunities in retirement, housing, retirement locations, health, legal affairs, financial planning, and adjustment to changes in lifestyles. Older people have the opportunity not only to learn from their participation but to train themselves to conduct PREP seminars.

Publications: The AOP offers materials and manuals for participation in and leadership of seminars across the country.

Active Corps of Executives   ACE
Suite 410
1129 20th Street, NW
Washington, DC 20036

(202) 653-6279

Profile: Active Corps of Executives is composed mainly of men and women who are retired and who volunteer to help people who are managing, or intending to manage, their own small businesses. At no cost for their time and expertise, ACE participants meet with the owners or managers of small businesses to advise them on ways to improve their efficiency, develop larger incomes, or avoid problems. Many of the people served by ACE are retirees who have started new businesses, whether for economic reasons or to avoid the boredom of retirement.

Administration on Aging   **AOA**
USDHHS
Office of Human Development Services
330 Independence Avenue, SW
Washington, DC 20201

(202) 245-0641

Profile: The AOA acts as an advocate for the elderly, studying legislation and programs affecting older people and taking steps to protect the rights of this constituency. The AOA serves as the principal agency for implementing programs of the Older Americans Act, which was enacted in 1967 to provide older Americans with opportunities for full participation in the benefits of our society. Such benefits include the best possible physical and mental health, suitable housing, employment without age discrimination, independence, and the availability of participation in civic, cultural, and recreational activities. The AOA can provide information on actions taken and proposed that are helpful to older people.

Publications: Papers and reports are available on these, and other, objectives and programs in progress.

Adult Development and Aging   **ADA**
Division 20
American Psychological Association
University of Missouri
Columbia, MO 65211

(314) 882-6389

Profile: The ADA is a professional society of psychologists who counsel people who are aging and have mental, emotional, or behavioral problems. Through the American Psychological Association, it offers continuing education programs, based on extensive research and investigation in this field.

Services: Through state chapters, the ADA helps individuals, couples, and families locate professional assistance for consultation and treatment.

Publications: Psychology Today (monthly) and *Psychology and Aging* (quarterly).

Adult Education Association of USA   **AEA**
1201 16th Street, NW
Washington, DC 20006

(202) 822-7866

Profile: The AEA is an independent, nonprofit organization dedicated to increasing and improving adult education programs in the United States. It supports research on education, sponsors seminars and workshops, and promotes enrollment in AEA-accredited programs. Inquiries are invited.

Publications: The AEA publishes professional periodicals on adult education, produces a directory of programs and affiliates, and distributes booklets on request.

AFL-CIO
Community Services Department
Suite 704
815 16th Street, NW
Washington, DC 20006

(202) 637-5000

Profile: The Community Services Department of the American Federation of Labor assists older people in the work force and also helps them in planning retirement and obtaining proper pensions and retirement benefits.

Aging in America   **AIA**
1500 Pelham Parkway
Bronx, NY 10461

(212) 824-4004

Profile: AIA was founded in 1979 as a research and service center for professionals in gerontology. Its objectives are to research and develop affordable programs and services that improve the quality of life for older people. Its educational and training programs are meaningful to older people wherever they are established. Examples of such programs are: Meals-on-Wheels, Alzheimer's day care centers, transportation for people who cannot drive or do not have the means, housekeeping for shut-ins, and social events for retirees.

Publications: Aging in America, newsletters, reports, and program curricula.

Aging Network Services   ANS
Suite 907
4400 East West Highway
Bethesda, MD 20814

(301) 657-4329

Profile: The ANS is a nonprofit nationwide network of social
workers in private practice who specialize in problems of retirees
and the elderly. They serve, too, as care managers for people who
live apart from their adult children.

Services: Through the ANS, retirees are better able to bridge the
distances between family members, remain independent, and
maintain better communications with relatives and friends. The
ANS arranges also for personal assistance with daily living
requirements, such as shopping, housekeeping, transportation,
and medical appointments.

Publications: Brochures describing services of the ANS.

Airline Passenger Association   APA
4301 Westside Drive
Dallas, TX 75209

(214) 520-1070

Profile: This organization was established as one to which travelers could turn for general information about air travel in the
United States and abroad. One section is devoted to travel information and counsel for people who are older, infirm, or handicapped.

Publications: Booklets about airline services, routes, and assistance programs for those in need.

Airline Passenger Complaints
Office of Intergovernmental
and Consumer Affairs
Department of Transportation
400 7th Avenue, SW
Washington, DC 20590

(202) 366-2220

Profile: This unit of the Department of Transportation was established in order to keep records of complaints about airlines and air travel and take remedial action. It is specially sensitive and responsive to complaints of older people and the problems they experienced that have not been resolved by individual airlines. People with such complaints, however, are urged to contact this agency only if they cannot receive satisfaction from the airline on which they have traveled.

Alcoholics Anonymous   **AA**
Box 459, Grand Central Station
New York, NY 10163

(212) 686-1100

Profile: AA is recognized as the most widespread and generally most successful program for helping people to recover from alcoholism. Founded in 1935, AA has developed a philosophy of life that has made it possible for countless millions of people to give up drinking and lead more normal, productive lives. The organization functions through local groups, which can be located in almost every town in the United States simply by looking up "AA" in the phone book and asking for information and assistance. Although AA has been successful with every age group, it can be particularly effective for retirees and older people at a stage in their lives when many tend to drink more than they used to or are no longer able to drink without problems.

Publications: AA publishes a number of books and many pamphlets on drinking, all emphasizing what AA can do to help alcoholics.

Alliance for Aging Research   **AAR**
Suite 305
2021 K Street, NW
Washington, DC 20006

(202) 293-2856

Profile: The AAR is a private, nonprofit organization dedicated to the promotion and support of research on the process of human aging and related matters. It serves as a clearinghouse of information and conducts educational programs to increase understanding and communication between agencies and associations that serve retirees and other older people. The AAR also lobbies for additional funding for research that will benefit older people and address the problems of aging.

Communications: The AAR publishes quarterly reports on its activities, which are available to anyone interested, and also conducts national print and broadcast media campaigns to inform the public about the need for research on aging.

Alliance to Save Energy   **ASE**
1925 K Street, NW, #206
Washington, DC 20006

(202) 857-0666

Profile: The ASE is a group of energy-related organizations whose joint goal is to research ways to save energy and advise the public. Seniors who want information about energy saving, or sources of further data, should contact the ASE.

Alternative Living for the Aging   **ALA**
937 North Fairfax Avenue
West Hollywood, CA 90046

(213) 650-7988

Profile: The ALA is a nonprofit organization whose objective is to provide housing alternatives for older people who otherwise might have to live alone or enter an institution. For those interested, the ALA can suggest innovative ways for older people to share their lives and yet retain privacy, dignity, and independence. The ALA is also active in supporting legislation that will enhance the housing situation for older Americans.

Alzheimer's Disease   **ADRDA**
and Related Disorders Association
Suite 600
70 East Lake Street
Chicago, IL 60601

(312) 853-3060
(800) 621-0379

Profile: This association is a voluntary agency dedicated to research into the cause, treatment, and cure for Alzheimer's disease. It supports local groups, provides technical assistance to governmental agencies, conducts training programs, and provides information for individuals and families who are concerned about this debilitating disease.

Publications: The ADRDA distributes publications that describe Alzheimer's, the current status of research, and methods for preventing and treating the disease.

Alzheimer's Disease   **ADEAR**
Education and Referral Center
PO Box 8250
Silver Spring, MD 20907-8250

(301) 495-3311

Profile: ADEAR is a special service of the National Institute on Aging (see page 235) whose objective is to distribute information about Alzheimer's disease to professionals, patients and their families, and the general public.

Services: The center responds to inquiries from individuals by providing verbal or printed information about the disease and its diagnosis and treatment. It also maintains computerized data available through libraries and other referral sources.

Publications: ADEAR publishes and/or distributes literature about Alzheimer's disease and related problems. A catalog of these publications is available on request.

Amateur Golfer's Association   **AGAA**
of America
2843 Pembroke Road
Hollywood, FL 33020

(305) 921-0881

Profile: The mission of the AGAA is to promote interest in golf as a sport and to sponsor research to increase and improve golf courses and schools in the United States. It publishes lists of courses and sources of information and actively encourages participation by retired men and women.

Amateur Softball   **ASAA**
Association of America
2801 Northeast 50th Street
Oklahoma City, OK 73111

(405) 424-5266

Profile: The ASAA was formed in order to promote the sport of softball in the United States and provide interested people with the means for joining or organizing softball teams. There has been increasing interest among retirees in this sport.

American Academy of Dermatology   **AAD**
PO Box 1661
1567 Maple Avenue
Evanston, IL 60204-1661

(312) 869-3954

Profile: The AAD is a professional body of dermatologists, physicians who specialize in the diagnosis and treatment of skin diseases. In addition to offering continuing education and programs for these specialists, the AAD also provides the general public with information—both general and specific—about skin diseases, such as cancer, allergies and other irritating conditions, and skin care. The AAD is responsive to older people who write or phone for information or who need help in locating dermatologists in their areas.

Communications: The AAD produces audiovisual materials, bibliographies, and literature for professionals, but also publishes booklets on skin diseases and skin care for the general public.

American Academy   **AAFP**
of Family Physicians
1740 West 92nd Street
Kansas City, MO 64114-2756

(816) 333-9700

Profile: The AAFP is a professional organization of general practitioners ("family doctors"), established so that members could learn from each other and establish rules of conduct and procedure that would be beneficial to doctors and patients alike. In addition to providing member programs, AAFP maintains a widespread communications program for the public, providing information and materials on medicine and health care. A special Committee on Aging addresses itself to the medical and health problems of older people and distributes information accordingly, upon request. Individuals are also encouraged to contact the academy to locate family doctors when they move to new communities.

Publications: The AAFP publishes *The American Family Physician* monthly, and also produces brochures, films, and medical exhibits of interest to individuals and families.

American Academy of Neurology   **AAN**
Suite 335
2221 University Avenue, SE
Minneapolis, MN 55414

(612) 623-8115

Profile: The AAN is a professional organization of doctors and health professionals who specialize in researching, diagnosing, and treating disorders of the nervous system. It not only provides educational programs and services for members but maintains strong communications with the general public on subjects relating to its field. Individuals can contact the AAN for information about nervous disorders, or for assistance in locating specialists for consultation and treatment.

Publications: The AAN publishes a monthly journal, *Neurology,* and distributes informational pamphlets to the public on request.

American Academy of Ophthalmology   AAO
PO Box 7424
San Francisco, CA 94120-7424

(415) 561-8500
(800) 222-3973

Profile: The membership of the AAO consists of doctors and other health professionals who specialize in the diagnosis and treatment of eye diseases. It maintains a toll-free National Eye Care Project Helpline, which can be reached at the 800 number listed above from 8:00 A.M. to 5:00 P.M., PST. Callers are put in touch with ophthalmologists in their areas who have volunteered to provide free or low-cost eye care to older people. Information on the prevention and treatment of eye problems is readily available to the general public through AAO services.

Publications: The AAO distributes literature on eye care upon request.

American Academy of   AAOS
Orthopedic Surgeons
222 South Prospect Avenue
Park Ridge, IL 60068

(312) 823-7186

Profile: The AAOS is a professional society whose members are doctors specializing in treating bones, joints, muscles, ligaments, and tendons. It provides information to the public about musculoskeletal problems in general and specific information about such subjects as implant artificial joints, preventing osteoporosis, and relieving pain caused by bursitis and arthritis. The AAOS also maintains information for older people about diseases and conditions to which they are particularly susceptible, and helps individuals locate qualified orthopedists in their areas.

Publications: The AAOS publishes and distributes free brochures covering a wide range of subjects related to its field. A list is available on request.

American Academy of   **AAPMR**
Physical Medicine and Rehabilitation
122 South Michigan Avenue
Chicago, IL 60603-6107

(312) 922-9366

Profile: This organization is composed of doctors and health professionals, such as therapists, nurses, and social workers, who specialize in rehabilitation and whose objectives are to help individuals restore functions that have been impaired because of illness or injury. Special programs are dedicated to the problems and needs of older people who might require rehabilitative treatment. The AAPMR serves as an information clearinghouse for professionals and the public alike, and will assist individuals in locating specialists in their areas.

Publications: Publications are mainly for professional use, but the AAPMR suggests, and in some cases distributes, literature suitable for laypersons.

American Allergy Association
PO Box 7273
Menlo Park, CA 94026

(818) 991-6740

Profile: The members of this association are doctors or health specialists concerned with the identification and treatment of allergies of all kinds. Many such allergies affect older people, particularly those who move from one environment to another that is quite different. The association conducts and supports research on diet, environment, genealogy, working conditions, and other factors that cause or aggravate allergies.

Publications: The association publishes a newsletter and distributes literature on allergies upon request.

American Alliance for Health,   **AAHPERD**
Physical Education, Recreation, and Dance
1900 Association Drive
Reston, VA 22091

(703) 476-3461

Profile: The American Alliance is a nonprofit organization of more than thirty thousand professional educators in the fields of physical education, fitness, health, athletics, recreation, dance, and related disciplines. Founded in 1885, the alliance maintains the same goals it had more than a century ago: to improve the health and fitness of Americans through ongoing educational programs. An important category of activity relates to programs for people who are older, who are retiring, or who are changing locations and lifestyles.

Services: The AAHPERD provides information about the many activities with which it is involved and will suggest contacts and programs in individuals' own locations.

American Amateur   **AARA**
Racquetball Association
Suite 203
815 North Weber Street
Colorado Springs, CO 80903

(303) 635-5396

Profile: The AARA is composed of individuals and groups interested in promoting racquetball as a sport and developing improved facilities and programs. Older people interested in knowing more about the sport or organizing their own groups should write or phone the AARA for more information.

American Arbitration Association   **AAA**
140 West 51st Street
New York, NY 10020

(212) 484-4000

Profile: The American Arbitration Association, founded in 1926, is the country's leading private, nonprofit organization specializing in arbitrating and resolving disputes. It conducts studies in its subject field, maintains thirty-five offices nationwide, and invites inquiries from individuals and groups. The AAA can assist older people, or groups they belong to, in resolving business and consumer disputes without going to court.

Publications: The AAA distributes consumer literature on topics relating to the resolution of disputes and the avoidance of court and legal procedures.

American Association for   **AACC**
Continuity of Care
Suite 700
1101 Connecticut Avenue, NW
Washington, DC 20036

(202) 857-1100

Profile: The members of the AACC are largely organizations whose purpose is to provide long-term care and assistance to the elderly and the disabled. The association invites inquiries from older people who may need such care or from their families and dependents and will provide sources of more detailed or localized information.

American Association for   **AAIA**
International Aging
1511 K Street, NW
Washington, DC 20005

(202) 638-6815

Profile: The AAIA is a private, nonprofit organization established in 1983 in response to the Plan of Action on Aging prepared by the United Nations World Assembly on Aging. Members are organizations concerned with the needs of senior citizens in all countries of the world.

Publications: The AAIA publishes a newsletter, *Reports,* which highlights events of interest to senior citizens throughout the world.

American Association   **AABC**
of Backgammon Clubs
PO Box 12359
Las Vegas, NV 89119

(702) 388-2943

Profile: This association is active in promoting backgammon and helping people to organize groups and clubs to play the game. It welcomes the interest of retired people, many of whom are dedicated to backgammon.

American Association   **AAFS**
of Foot Specialists
PO Box 54
Union, NJ 07083

(201) 688-1616

Profile: The association's membership consists of podiatrists and other professionals who specialize in the diagnosis, care, and treatment of ailments and injuries relating to the feet. The AAFS conducts and supports research and develops educational programs for members. It also provides information on foot care for the general public and responds to specific inquiries about foot-related medical problems. Individuals can write or phone for references to podiatrists and other specialists in their areas.

Publications: The AAFS distributes literature on foot care, injuries, and disorders.

American Association of   **AAHA**
Homes for the Aging
Suite 500
901 E Street, NW
Washington, DC 20004-2837

(202) 783-2242

Profile: Founded in 1961, the AAHA is an organization of non-profit nursing homes, independent housing facilities, continuing care communities, and community service agencies. It provides a unified means for identifying and solving problems in order to protect and advance the interests of the residents served in these facilities. Its objectives include measures to help members meet the social, environmental, and health needs of the occupants and public education programs to encourage the community to become involved in enhancing and improving care and facilities alike. The AAHA provides information and counsel at no cost to individuals and families interested in homes and communities for older people.

Publications: The association publishes a number of periodicals, including *AAHA Provider News,* a biannual *Continuing Care Directory,* and a catalog of consumer publications that is available free of charge. A guidebook, *The Continuing Care Retirement Community,* is available from the AAHA for $4.00.

American Association of   **AAPHD**
Public Health Dentistry
10619 Jousting Lane
Richmond, VA 23235

(804) 786-3556

Profile: The AAPHD is composed of dentists and dental groups whose mission is to promote better dental and mouth care among people who rely on public-health services for health and medical needs and whose budgets are limited. Retirees and other older people with limited funds who are concerned about the high cost of dentistry, dentures, and related services should contact the AAPHD for information on dentistry available to them at little or no expense.

American Association   **AARP**
of Retired Persons
1909 K Street, NW
Washington, DC 20049

(202) 872-4880

Profile: AARP is a nonprofit, nonpartisan association dedicated to helping older people be independent and lead fruitful and digni-fied lives. Membership is open to anyone fifty or older, whether working or retired. The association offers a wide range of services and programs for older people and is active in proposing and sup-porting legislative measures at all governmental levels that will benefit this age group. Programs cover such subject areas as retirement, health, financial matters, legal affairs, housing, trans-portation, insurance, communication, family relationships, recre-ation, travel, adult education, and volunteer participation.

Publications: Membership in AARP includes subscriptions to the monthly newsletter, the bimonthly magazine *Modern Maturity,* and reports on subjects of special interest. AARP also offers a large variety of informative publications at little or no cost, and a wide range of full-length books. (Some of the latter are listed in the Bibliography of this guidebook). Audiovisual materials are also available on such subjects as health, employment, housing, lifelong learning, safety, crime prevention, women's issues, and consumer information.

**AARP Home Equity
Information Center**
Box A
1909 K Street, NW
Washington, DC 20049

(202) 872-4880

Profile: The Home Equity Branch of AARP focuses on the use of one's residence as a means of providing income for later retirement. Regular members of AARP can obtain general and specific information through queries to AARP or through the purchase of publications on this subject.

Publications: In addition to regular reports, AARP publishes a number of handbooks, including *Home-Made Money, Borrowing against Your Home,* and conversion fact sheets.

AARP Legal Counsel   **LCE**
for the Elderly
1909 K Street, NW
Washington, DC 20049

(202) 872-4880

Profile: The LCE division of AARP is dedicated to assisting older
people in handling legal matters of many kinds, from the routine
to the critical, and in the use of reliable counsel when necessary.
To this end, AARP also conducts investigations into conditions
and circumstances that affect older people from a legal point of
view and recommends methods for avoiding or minimizing legal
problems.

Publications: Among the many publications on legal topics available to members are ones about law enforcement, personal
rights, lawsuits, housing regulations and restrictions, fighting
fraud, and the preparation of wills and other legal instruments.

AARP Worker Equity Department
1909 K Street, NW
Washington, DC 20049

(202) 662-4958

Profile: In 1984, AARP made a decision to focus its resources on
efforts to aid older workers, to help them prepare for retirement
and career changes, and to protect them from age discrimination
in the workplace. To fulfill this pledge, AARP established the
Worker Equity Initiative, a program designed to achieve cooperation with and procure benefits from organizations who hire, or
might hire, older people. AARP members are thus able to benefit
from the breakthroughs achieved, as well as through communications that provide information of particular interest to them.

Publications: Available to AARP members are publications on job-related subjects such as safety, pension rights, worker equity programs, options for women, and preretirement planning.

American Automobile Association   **AAA**
8111 Gatehouse Road
Falls Church, VA 22047

(703) 222-6446

Profile: The American Automobile Association has been a particular boon to older motorists because its services are designed to enhance trips of any length, improve the safety of drivers and passengers, minimize traffic inconveniences, and provide quick, reliable emergency service twenty-four hours a day, seven days a week, around the calendar. These include jump-starting when batteries are dead; changing flat tires; towing; extricating vehicles from mud, snow, and ditches; gaining entry when owners are locked out; and providing basic assistance in case of accidents. Over the years, AAA has broadened its services to include many related functions, such as insurance, credit cards, travel services, tours, loans, discounts on accommodations and meals, bail bonds, and theft protection.

Publications: AAA provides maps and tour guides tailored to individual needs, newsletters, a magazine, and an abundance of literature about highways and byways, accommodations, services, and just about every facet of travel by car, plane, train, or boat.

American Bankers Association   **ABA**
Personal Economics Program
1120 Connecticut Avenue NW
Washington, DC 20006

(202) 663-5470

Profile: The ABA is the national trade and professional association for America's full-service banks, representing about 95 percent of the banking industry. It serves as a lobbying organization to promote legislation beneficial to its members and the banking public, sponsors seminars and workshops, and produces literature for professionals and consumers.

Publications: The ABA distributes booklets, releases, and fact sheets on topics of interest to consumers, including checking and savings accounts, home equity loans, mortgages, auto financing, credit cards, credit ratings, and retirement budgets.

American Bed and Breakfast Association   **ABBA**
Suite 203
16 Village Green
Crofton, MD 21114

(301) 261-0180

Profile: Members of ABBA are for the most part private citizens who are proprietors of rooms they have made available, in their own homes or adjoining structures, for the use of motorists. Older travelers have found them appealing because of their modest rates, friendly atmospheres, quiet environments, and hearty fare. ABBA serves as a clearinghouse for information about B&B locations and accommodations in the United States, most of North America, and in some cases abroad. The association sponsors an Evergreen Bed and Breakfast Club, which offers lower rates and discounts for travelers over fifty.

Publications: ABBA provides published lists and rates for its members, along with basic information of interest to travelers. ABBA, though not a sponsor, has also contributed reliable data for a number of book-length guides on B&Bs.

American Bowling Congress   **ABC**
5301 South 76th Street
Greendale, WI 53129

(414) 421-6400

Profile: The members of the American Bowling Congress are individuals and professionals interested in promoting bowling as a family recreation and a competitive sport for all ages. It maintains directories of bowling alleys and clubs, sponsors lessons and workshops, and focuses one segment of its programs on the advantages of bowling for older people. Inquiries are encouraged.

American Bridge Association   **ABA**
555 Kapock Street #12G
Riverdale, NY 10463

(212) 543-2911

Profile: The work of the ABA is largely directed to programs involving competition, rules, and the planning of tournaments and other major bridge events. However, the ABA encourages inquiries from older people interested in learning more about the game, taking courses, and getting involved. It provides references to local sources of information.

American Cancer Society   **ACS**
1599 Clifton Road, NE
Atlanta, GA 30329

(404) 320-3333

Also:
1825 Connecticut Avenue, NW
Washington, DC 10009

(202) 483-2600
Hotline: (800) 227-2345

Profile: The American Cancer Society is a voluntary, nonprofit agency whose basic objective is to obtain and direct funds for cancer research, as well as to educate the public about cancer prevention, detection, and treatment. Local ACS chapters sponsor a wide range of services for cancer patients and their families, including self-help groups. Special programs are designed for older people who have cancer or are highly susceptible to it; other programs help patients meet the physical, cosmetic, and emotional needs related to the disease.

Publications: The ACS offers numerous free publications on all forms of cancer, as well as literature containing general information about cancer prevention, detection, and treatment. Such publications are available from the national office in Atlanta or from local offices listed in phone directories nationwide.

American Center for   **ACHPA**
Health Promotion and Aging
National Council on Aging (NCOA)
West Wing 100
600 Maryland Avenue, SW
Washington, DC 20024

(202) 479-1200

Profile: The ACHPA is a nonprofit membership organization for medical and health professionals who are concerned with the health and well-being of older people. The center serves as a clearinghouse for information, as well as a catalyst for obtaining funds and promoting research on the relationships between aging and health. The ACHPA serves as an advocate on behalf of older persons and helps sponsor programs and legislation to meet their continuing health needs. Older individuals can obtain data and information about such programs at no cost, as well as references to sources and materials of particular interest.

Publications: The ACHPA and the NCOA publish a number of periodicals, including *Perspectives on Aging* and *Senior Center Report.* Numerous brochures are available upon request on topics of interest to seniors.

American Chess Foundation   **ACF**
Box 15
Whitestone, NY 11357

(212) 353-1456

Profile: This organization consists largely of people who are serious and dedicated chess players interested in competition and other organizations involved with the game. The ACF can provide interested people with referrals to local groups in their areas and sources of further information.

American College of Physicians   ACP
Suite 425
655 15th Street, NW
Washington, DC 20005

(202) 393-1650
(800) 523-1546

Profile: The ACP is a professional society of internists who treat diseases in adults. Many members specialize in fields pertinent to the health of older people, such as cardiology, infectious diseases, rheumatology, disorders of the digestive system, and cancer. The college sponsors scientific meetings, conducts seminars, and maintains a constantly updated system of communication to keep the medical profession and the public informed. Although the thrust of ACP activities is toward the professional, the college encourages members to make current information about medicine and health available to the patients they serve.

Communications: In addition to professional periodicals, the ACP produces *Healthscope,* a film series that acquaints laypersons with the symptoms and treatments of various diseases.

American College of Surgeons   ACS
55 East Erie Street
Chicago, IL 60611

(312) 664-4050

Profile: The American College of Surgeons is an organization whose members are accredited surgeons; its major objective is to ensure that all surgical patients receive the finest possible treatment and care. The college offers continuing programs to educate members about the latest techniques, equipment, and technology in their field. It also reaches out to the public with programs designed to inform them about the nature of new surgical methods and after-care, ways to rate hospital services, and the advisibility of second opinions when facing major surgery. The special needs of older patients are expressly addressed in many of these communications.

Publications: In addition to professional periodicals, the ACS also publishes and distributes educational materials on different kinds of surgery, convalescence, and costs.

American Contract Bridge League   **ACBL**
2200 Democrat Road
Memphis, TN 38116

(901) 332-5586

Profile: The work of the ACBL is largely directed to programs involving competition, rules, the planning of tournaments, and the furtherance of contract bridge. But the league does respond to inquiries from beginners interested in learning more about the game and provides references to local sources of further information.

American Council of Life Insurance   **ACLI**
1001 Pennsylvania Avenue, NW
Washington, DC 20004-2599

(202) 624-2414

Profile: The membership of the ACLI consists of more than six hundred companies that account for 95 percent of the life insurance business. The council is readily accessible to retirees and other older people who have questions about life insurance and related matters. It can also provide information or suggest sources for data concerning such subjects as death benefits for survivors, mandatory health care programs, and the facts about mail-order insurance and television commercials touting life insurance for older people with no physical examination required.

Publications: The ACLI publishes and/or distributes numerous brochures and fact sheets on insurance. Subjects covered also include health care choices, Medicare, Medicare supplemental coverage, long-term care, and community support groups.

American Council of the Blind   **ACB**
Suite 1100
1010 Vermont Avenue, NW
Washington, DC 20005

(202) 393-3666
(800) 424-8666

Profile: The ACB is a nonprofit organization whose basic objective is to improve the lifestyle of people who are blind or whose vision is seriously impaired. The council serves as an advocate for better health care, Social Security benefits, and facilities for visually impaired people, both within their communities and while traveling. The ACB hotline, the 800 number given above, is accessible weekdays from 3:00 P.M. to 5:00 P.M., EST, to provide callers with information and take requests for literature.

Communications: Braille Forum is published bimonthly and distributed free to the blind, the visually impaired, and sighted persons who are specially interested. It is available in braille, large print, and audiocassette, as are numerous other ACB productions.

American Council on Alcoholism   **ACA**
8501 LaSalle Road
Towson, MD 21204

(301) 296-5555

Profile: The mission of the ACA, a private, nonprofit organization, is to educate the public about the disease of alcoholism, its prevention, and treatment. It distributes information through several media to professionals and consumers alike, promotes the establishment of local affiliates to combat alcoholism, and supports research into the causes and effects of excessive drinking. Technical assistance is provided to community organizations that provide assistance to alcoholics and their families. Special attention is also focused on alcoholism that develops in older people and its effects on them. The ACA responds to inquiries and makes referrals to local groups and treatment facilities.

Communications: The ACA produces and distributes numerous free booklets on alcoholism and related subjects. It also makes available, or refers people to sources of, films, cassettes, and other audiovisual material that can be borrowed or rented.

American Craft Council   **ACC**
40 West 53rd Street
New York, NY 10019

(212) 956-3535

Profile: Members of the ACC are individuals, groups, clubs, and businesspeople interested in furthering the interest of the American public in crafts, particularly those that are native to the country's various regions. The council provides information about craft-related events, courses, and local contacts for people interested in specific types of crafts. Particular attention is given to retired people who are seeking new hobbies and leisure-time pursuits.

American Dental Association   **ADA**
Department of Public Information
211 East Chicago Avenue
Chicago, IL 60611

(312) 440-2500

Profile: The ADA is a professional organization whose members are dedicated to improving the dental health of the public and promoting the art and science of dentistry. The association maintains continuing seminars on dental research and procedures, encourages members to participate in community outreach programs to communicate with the public, and helps to establish low-cost (sometimes free) dental services for older people. The ADA can also help individuals locate the right dentist for their needs when they move to a new community.

Publications: Special Care in Dentistry is published bimonthly by the ADA. Information for older people about planning their dental programs is also available. The ADA distributes free materials on tooth decay, dentures, and other aspects of mouth care.

American Dental Hygienist's Association   ADHA

Suite 3400
444 North Michigan Avenue
Chicago, IL 60611

(312) 440-8900

Profile: The ADHA is composed of dental specialists whose objectives are to improve the dental health of the people they serve. Special programs are aimed at communicating with older people about their specific kinds of needs, particularly the preparation and use of dentures and bridges. ADHA members participate in community training programs relating to the proper care of the teeth.

Publications: Literature is available at no cost from the ADHA on such subjects as cleaning the teeth and gums, selecting proper toothbrushes, flossing, removing plaque, and the prevention of gum disease.

American Diabetes Association   ADA

1660 Duke Street
Alexandria, VA 22314

(703) 549-1500
(800) 232-3472

Profile: The ADA is a voluntary, nonprofit organization that encourages and supports research to cure and treat diabetes. Its other major objectives are to improve the understanding and well-being of diabetic patients and their families, educate the public about the warning symptoms of the disease, provide first-hand information about its diagnosis and prompt treatment, and make known the resources available for people with diabetes.

Programs are provided by local chapters of the ADA, many of them focusing on the problems and needs of older people who are, or might become, diabetic. The ADA also helps individuals and families select specialists.

Publications: The association publishes a number of periodicals for its members, covering research and development in this field. It also distributes useful pamphlets to the public, including *Diabetes in the Family, Diabetes: Reach for Health and Freedom,* and *The Family Cookbook.*

American Dietetic Association   **ADA**
Suite 800
216 West Jackson Boulevard
Chicago, IL 60606-6995

(312) 899-0400

Profile: The American Dietetic Association is a professional society of some fifty thousand dieticians who work in schools, centers for older people, day care facilities, and commercial and industrial establishments. They provide counseling on nutrition, health, and the prevention of illnesses caused by improper diet. The association offers continuing education programs for its members, as well as the public at large. One group of dieticians is assigned to a program known as Area Agencies on Aging, which devotes itself to Meals-on-Wheels, home health agencies, and other health-care programs that meet the special nutritional needs of older people. Members also provide counseling to older people and can help them in locating proper facilities and professional assistance.

Publications: The association publishes two professional journals and distributes pamphlets on nutrition and diet to the public upon request.

American Federation   **AFAR**
for Aging Research
725 Park Avenue
New York, NY 10021

(212) 570-2090

Profile: The AFAR's objectives are to encourage and support basic and clinical biomedical research in the field of aging, and to develop public support for research in this field. Funds support studies on the physiological and psychological aspects of aging, genetics, human growth and development, lifestyle and environmental factors and their relationships with growing older, and diseases that produce disabilities or affect life span.

Publications: The AFAR produces professional journals, but also makes available a list of publications of interest to the general public and particularly to older people.

American Financial Services Association   **AFSA**
1101 14th Street, NW
Washington, DC 20005

(202) 289-0400
(800) 843-3280

Profile: The AFSA is an organization whose objective is to assist the public in personal and private economic matters. Among the continuing studies made by the AFSA are ones relating to the financial problems and needs of retirees. The AFSA promotes the business of direct credit lending to consumers and provides information for individuals and families on money management and the use of credit.

Publications: Retirees and other older people can obtain consumer budget guides and other such literature produced by the AFSA upon request.

American Foundation for the Blind   **AFB**
15 West 16th Street
New York, NY 10011

(212) 620-2147
(800) 232-5463

Also:
1660 L Street, NW
Washington, DC 20036

(202) 467-5996

Profile: This nonprofit foundation consists of members who develop programs and provide services to assist people who are blind or visually impaired, with the intent of making them more independent and self-sufficient. The AFB works with specialized schools and agencies throughout the country to develop educational programs and provide consumer products and materials for this audience. The AFB maintains a toll-free hotline, the 800 number given above, which is available weekdays from 8:30 A.M. to 4:30 P.M., EST, to respond to questions about products and services. The foundation also records Talking Books for the Library of Congress.

Communications: Through the above offices and regional offices, the AFB makes available a wide range of publications in braille, large print, and audiocassette. A catalog is available at no cost upon request.

American Geriatrics Society   **AGS**
Suite 400
770 Lexington Avenue
New York, NY 10021

(212) 308-1414

Profile: Founded in 1942, the AGS is a professional society of doctors and others concerned with the health care of older people and the research directed toward its advancement. The society promotes training in geriatric medicine and stresses the importance of medical research in the field of aging. The AGS communicates with the general public, especially older people, on such topics as geriatric medicine, long- and short-term care, acute and chronic illnesses, rehabilitation, and nursing homes. Individuals are encouraged to contact the society for help in locating geriatricians (specialists in aging) or to obtain information about specific medical problems.

Publications: The AGS publishes a journal and newsletter and also distributes pamphlets and reports at no cost to individuals concerned about this field of medicine and health.

American Health Care Association   **AHCA**
1201 L Street, NW
Washington, DC 20005

(202) 842-4444

Profile: The AHCA is a nonprofit federation of associations in fifty states and the District of Columbia that serve some 9,500 licensed nursing homes and allied facilities. The association provides leadership in dealing with long-term care facilities, and offers continuing education programs for nursing home professionals. For the consumer, the AHCA provides educational materials on long-term care and (through its main office and regional offices) answers questions from individuals and families about available facilities and programs in their areas.

Publications: Booklets on selecting a nursing home, guardianship, long-term care service, and other pertinent subjects in this field are readily available to the public.

American Health Planning Association   **AHPA**
Suite 950
1110 Vermont Avenue, NW
Washington, DC 20005

(202) 861-1200

Profile: One of the missions of the AHPA is to help older people and their families plan for long-term health care, both in the home and in institutions. It provides inquirers with background data, directories, and referrals to sources of local information.

American Health Foundation   **AHF**
320 East 43rd Street
New York, NY 10017

(212) 953-1900

Profile: The American Health Foundation, a private, nonprofit agency, conducts research in preventive medicine and studies the relationships between age, lifestyle, environment, nutrition, and other factors in the development of cancer and other major diseases. The AHF investigates ways in which normal cells become cancerous, identifies cancer-causing substances, and conducts projects involving health promotion and disease prevention in older individuals.

Publications: The AHF publishes *Health Letter* and *Preventive Medicine* for paid subscribers and distributes a *Health Passport,* which includes guidelines for preventing heart disease and cancer and can be used by individuals to maintain an annual health record.

American Heart Association   **AHA**
7320 Greenville Avenue
Dallas, TX 75231

(214) 373-6300

Profile: As one of the best known voluntary nonprofit organizations, the American Heart Association sponsors widespread public-education programs to help reduce premature death and disability from heart attack, stroke, and other heart and blood-vessel diseases. The AHA distributes free materials on the prevention and control of diseases of the heart and circulatory system, acquires research funds, and encourages many local programs and projects in this field. Local chapters, for example, sponsor stroke clubs, where patients and families exchange practical information about illness and recovery, and where specialists speak on heart-related subjects. The AHA also sponsors group efforts to eliminate smoking.

Publications: A list of publications is available from AHA headquarters or local chapters. These include booklets and brochures on heart disease, strokes, and *An Older Person's Guide to Cardiovascular Health.*

American Hiking Society   **AHS**
1701 18th Street, NW
Washington, DC 20009

(202) 234-4609

Profile: The American Hiking Society was founded to promote greater public interest in walking and hiking as a healthful form of exercise. The society regularly communicates information to the public about hiking trails, in-city walking routes, walking and hiking clubs, and the physical and psychological benefits of moving on one's feet.

Publications: The society distributes free literature on walking and hiking and suggests relevant books and periodicals that are available at varying costs.

American Home Economics Association   **AHEA**
2010 Massachusetts Avenue, NW
Washington, DC 20036

(202) 862-8300

Profile: The American Home Economics Association is a nonprofit organization established to make all aspects of home economics and homemaking more efficient, enjoyable, and rewarding.

American Hospital Association   **AHA**
840 North Lake Shore Drive
Chicago, IL 60611

(312) 280-6000
(800) 242-2626

Profile: The American Hospital Association is a professional, non-profit organization representing hospitals and other facilities that provide residential and outpatient medical care. The AHA offers continuing education programs for hospital administrators, maintains a health-administration library, and distributes information to the public on the many aspects of hospital care. To help hospitals meet the special needs of older patients, the Office on Aging and Long-Term Care conducts research in fields affecting seniors and helps to coordinate the activities of other community organizations that provide health services to these people.

Publications: Among numerous publications of interest to older laypersons are *A Patient's Bill of Rights, The Hospital's Role in Caring for the Elderly,* and the *AHA Catalog.*

American Institute of   **AICPA**
Certified Public Accountants
1211 Avenue of the Americas
New York, NY 10036

(212) 575-6209

Profile: The American Institute of Certified Public Accountants was established to help CPAs and other accounting specialists maintain standards and exchange information about accounting procedures, practices, and ethics. The AICPA maintains regular communications with the general public, informing individuals about the benefits of using CPAs for personal accounting and the maintenance of adequate records.

Publications: The AICPA distributes informational booklets and reports at no cost on a variety of pertinent topics. Of special interest to older people are those related to financial planning, taxes, estates, and trusts.

American Insurance Services Group   **AISG**
85 John Street
New York, NY 10038

(212) 669-0419

Profile: A subsidiary of the American Insurance Association, the AISG specializes in property casualty insurance. Of special interest to retirees and older people are studies determining better ways to develop claim settlement techniques, fight frauds, estimate casualty losses, and evaluate situations relating to claims regarding fire, home construction, environmental problems, product safety, and crime prevention.

Publications: The AISG distributes booklets at no cost on the above topics and many others.

American Liver Foundation   **ALF**
998 Pompton Avenue
Cedar Grove, NJ 07009

(201) 857-2626
(800) 223-0179

Profile: The American Liver Foundation was established to generate funds and support research on liver diseases, provide practical information for patients and their families, and promote public awareness of disease symptoms and treatments. The ALF also administers an ongoing program of organ donations for liver transplants, and responds to inquiries from private citizens about resources for treatment. Upon request, the ALF refers individuals to local specialists.

Publications: The AFL distributes free literature on such subjects as preventive measures, treatment, transplants, cirrhosis, and the relationship between heavy drinking and liver diseases.

American Lung Association   **ALA**
1740 Broadway
New York, NY 10019-4374

(212) 315-8700

Profile: The ALA is a voluntary, nonprofit organization whose purpose is to conduct educational programs on the prevention, detection, and treatment of lung diseases and on methods of living with disabled breathing. An important priority is the association's ongoing programs to discourage smoking. Also important is its program to educate the public about environmental and occupational hazards related to breathing and the lungs. The association readily makes available free information and counsel on the detection and treatment of lung ailments, which include cancer, chronic bronchitis, tuberculosis, and emphysema, among others.

Publications: In addition to publishing *The American Review of Respiratory Disease* for health professionals, the ALA produces numerous consumer publications, self-help guides, posters, and films on lung health. These are available through local chapters, which are listed in the telephone directory.

American Medical Association   **AMA**
535 North Dearborn Street
Chicago, IL 60610

(312) 751-6426

Profile: Best known of all medical associations, the AMA basically represents and protects the interests of physicians and maintains broad public relations programs to communicate its viewpoints to laypersons in every part of the country. The AMA distributes scientific data to health professionals of all kinds, as well as to the general public, informs doctors about significant legislation in their fields, and acts as a lobbying organization for the medical professional. It also coordinates its activities with other professional organizations in order to set better standards for private practice, hospitals, medical schools, and health educational facilities. Through state and local branches and related associations, the AMA provides physician referral services for the public and serves as an arbitrator in investigating medical complaints. The AMA maintains numerous services that are of special interest to retirees, other older people, and geriatric patients. Information on services and facilities can be obtained through local branches and affiliates of the AMA.

Publications: The AMA publishes a number of periodicals for the medical profession, produces informative pamphlets about medicine and health, and sponsors a number of guidebooks that are available at libraries and bookstores. Examples are: *The AMA Home Medical Advisor* and the *AMA Guide to Prescription and Over-the-Counter Drugs,* both published by Random House. For other books, see the Bibliography at the end of this resource guide.

American Mobilehome Association   **AHA**
12929 West 26th Avenue
Golden, CO 80401

(303) 232-6336

Profile: The American Mobilehome Association was founded by mobile-home owners as a means for exchanging information of mutual interest, lobbying for better recognition and treatment, and proposing legislation that would benefit members. Activities and subjects are of special interest to the large segment of mobile-home owners who are retirees.

Publications: The association publishes a monthly magazine, distributes brochures on mobile homes, and lists other publications that are pertinent to the field, such as *Tips on Buying a Mobile Home* (Council of Better Business Bureaus) and *How to Buy a Manufactured (Mobile) Home* (Consumer Information Center).

American Model Yachting Association   **AMYA**
104 West Lake Boulevard
Sebring, FL 33870

(813) 385-8529

Profile: Membership in the AMYA consists of individuals, clubs, and organizations interested in designing, making, and sailing model yachts, and, in appropriate locations, in racing competitions. Retired people whose hobby is model yacht making or sailing are encouraged to contact the AMYA for information about the association and model yachting events.

American Movers Conference   **AMC**
1611 Duke Street
Alexandria, VA 22314

(703) 683-7410

Profile: The AMC is the trade association of the interstate household goods moving industry, whose 1,750 members handle more than 90 percent of all interstate household moves. The AMC can be particularly helpful to older people who may be retiring and moving to new locations with which they are not totally familiar. The AMC works with the American Arbitration Association (see page 64) to settle any claims involving loss or damage to goods transported by AMC members. The AMC also communicates regularly with the public on subjects related to the moving of household goods and equipment.

Publications: The AMC prepares and distributes informational literature at no cost upon request. Examples are: *Guide to a Satisfying Move, Moving with Plants and Pets,* and *Moving and Children.*

American Natural Hygiene Society   **ANHS**
12816 Race Track Road
Tampa, FL 33625

(813) 855-6607

Profile: The ANHS is a nonprofit public-health education organization that concentrates on maintaining health through natural means, such as the consumption of natural foods, outdoor living, and the avoidance of environments that are polluted or otherwise harmful. The members of the society maintain an ongoing public relations campaign to inform consumers about matters that are beneficial— or injurious—to health. Many retirees and older people who have moved away from cities find an interest in this subject.

Publications: The ANHS produces a bimonthly magazine, books, tapes, and informative literature, available upon request.

American Newspaper   **ANPA**
Publishers Association
PO Box 17022
Dulles International Airport
Washington, DC 20041

(703) 648-1038

Profile: The ANPA represents newspaper publishers across the country and has long been a driving force in promoting newspapers as the number-one medium for reaching consumers. Consumers who are victims of fraud or distress as a result of any form of newspaper advertising are encouraged to contact the ANPA with their complaints. Many of these victims are retirees who have been conned into making shaky investments or shoddy purchases. Older people with complaints of any kind against newspapers have recourse through the ANPA if the complaint cannot be satisfactorily resolved through the newspaper involved.

American Nurses Association   **ANA**
2420 Pershing Road
Kansas City, MO 64108

(816) 474-5720

Profile: The ANA is the professional organization for registered nurses, representing some 185,000 members in fifty-three state associations. The ANA Council on Gerontological Nursing recommends and implements policies relating to health care for older adults. The association studies health care needs and practices and lobbies at state and federal levels for appropriate legislation to protect and improve nursing care. The ANA communicates regularly with consumers through various media to enhance public understanding of nursing and facilities.

Publications: The ANA publishes *The American Journal of Nursing* monthly and a newspaper, *American Nurse,* ten times a year. It also makes available a number of informative booklets, including *Facts about Nursing.* A list of other materials is available on request.

American Nursing Home Association   **ANHA**
Affiliate of American Health Care Association
1201 L Street, NW
Washington, DC 20005

(202) 842-4444

Profile: The American Nursing Home Association is committed to plans and programs that upgrade the standards in nursing homes, provide more reliable care, improve safety conditions, and coordinate activities with related medical and health groups. The ANHA has affiliates in all fifty states and refers phone calls and mail inquiries to local chapters.

Publications: The association distributes information on nursing homes to the general public and maintains a directory of accredited nursing homes throughout the United States and in parts of Canada.

American Philatelic Society   APS

PO Box 8000
State College, PA 16801

(814) 237-3803

Profile: The American Philatelic Society is composed largely of individuals who collect postage stamps, stamp clubs, and various firms that deal in these collectibles. The APS maintains lists of national and local sources of information, as well as stamp dealers and clubs.

American Physical Fitness   APFRI
Research Institute

654 North Sepulveda Boulevard
Los Angeles, CA 90049

(213) 426-6241

Profile: The institute is largely concerned with research into methods, programs, and equipment for developing and improving physical fitness of Americans of all ages. A considerable effort is aimed at ways and means to upgrade the fitness of older people, especially those who are retired or retiring and interested in maintaining better fitness and health. The institute responds to inquiries from the public.

American Physical Therapy Association   APTA

1111 North Fairfax Street
Alexandria, VA 22314

(703) 684-2782

Profile: An organization of health professionals, the APTA is committed to helping patients recover disabled functions following accident, injury, stroke, or other illness. Physical therapists are trained in the use of exercise, heat, water therapy, and other treatments to strengthen muscles and improve coordination. The APTA undertakes research and study programs in this field and maintains a special Geriatrics Section to assist older patients who face disabling conditions, such as acute arthritis, or who are recovering from a stroke or other critical illness. Members of the Geriatrics Section are also devoted to helping healthy older people remain fit.

Publications: The APTA distributes a number of informative booklets, such as *Take a Look at Today's Physical Therapist* and *Don't Become a Pain Statistic.*

American Podiatric Medical Association   **APMA**
9312 Old Georgetown Road
Bethesda, MD 20814

(301) 571-9200

Profile: The American Podiatric Medical Association is composed of doctors who specialize in diagnosing and treating injuries and diseases of the feet. The APMA promotes good foot care to the public in order to create a greater awareness of preventive measures that will avoid disorders and discomfort. One of the APMA's continuing projects relates to the degenerative process in older people and methods of minimizing foot problems caused by age.

Publications: The association publishes and distributes numerous free pamphlets to the public. Examples are: *Let's Talk about Foot Care and You, Your Podiatrist Talks about Foot Care and Aging,* and *Arthritis and Your Feet.*

American Printing House for the Blind   APHB

1839 Frankfort Avenue
Louisville, KY 40206-0085

(502) 895-2405

Profile: The American Printing House for the Blind is a private, nonprofit organization committed to the adaptation of books into braille for use by the blind and people with severely impaired vision.

Communications: The printing house offers a free catalog of materials for the blind and visually impaired. These include books and other publications in braille, braille writing and embossing equipment, electronic communications devices, low-vision simulation materials, and a variety of education aids.

American Psychiatric Association   APA

1400 K Street, NW
Washington, DC 20005

(202) 682-6000

Profile: The American Psychiatric Association is composed of psychiatrists and other medical doctors who specialize in diagnosing and treating patients with mental or emotional disorders. Among the APA's objectives are research to enhance the rehabilitation of disturbed patients, and programs to establish better standards for patient care, improved facilities, and continuing education. A special Council on Aging studies psychiatric care for older patients and those who are having trouble adjusting to their retirement. Particular attention is paid to ways to match patients with doctors to achieve favorable results.

Publications: Although APA publications are tailored mainly for doctors and other professionals, the association does distribute some literature that is informative for laypersons.

American Public Health Association   **APHA**
1015 15th Street, NW
Washington, DC 20005

(202) 789-5600

Profile: The APHA is composed largely of professionals and officials in the public health field whose mission is to increase and improve services throughout the United States. Although the APHA has few services of direct interest to consumers, it does provide directories of facilities and refers individuals to local sources of information and assistance.

American Public Welfare Association   **APWA**
1125 15th Street, NW
Washington, DC 20005

(202) 293-7550

Profile: The APWA was established as a nonprofit organization to study the administration of common public services, such as the distribution of food stamps, the maintenance of adequate incomes, and the processing of Medicare and Medicaid claims.

American Red Cross   **ARC**
National Headquarters
17th and D Streets, NW
Washington, DC 20006

(202) 737-8300

Profile: The American Red Cross provides numerous services of interest to older people, including health education programs, home nursing instruction, and blood processing and supply, all of which have been associated with the organization for many years. However, through local chapters, ARC also offers retirement planning, instruction in crime prevention, safety courses, shopper programs, telephone reassurance, health screening clinics, and visitation. Red Cross instructors teach courses on healthy life-styles, first aid, cardiopulmonary resuscitation (CPR), swimming, lifesaving, boating safety, and family health. Through the Program Exchange Process, a PEP catalog is published regularly that lists programs according to the activity and type of audience served.

Publications: Free pamphlets are available on a wide range of topics, including aging, diet, health, safety, and numerous illnesses and disabilities.

American Rheumatism Association   **ARA**
Suite 4809
17 Executive Park Drive
Atlanta, GA 30329

For information on rheumatism and related disorders, see the entry for the Arthritis Foundation, page 108.

American Running and   **ARFA**
Fitness Association
2001 S Street, NW
Washington, DC 20001

(202) 667-4150

Profile: The organization was founded to promote better health through running and other vigorous forms of exercise. The ARFA communicates with the general public through releases and reports that discuss running, walking, other forms of athletics, and ways to stay fit and trim and avoid illness. The association encourages inquiries from retirees who are interested in or have questions about fitness and preventive medicine.

Publications: The ARFA distributes publications in these subject areas and lists books and periodicals that are pertinent.

American Self-Help Clearinghouse

See the entry for the National Self-Help Clearinghouse, page 254.

American Senior Citizens Association   **ASCA**
PO Box 41
Fayetteville, NC 20302

(919) 323-3641

Profile: Founded in 1982, the ASCA is composed of some thirty-five thousand seniors whose purpose is to enhance their physical, mental, emotional, and economic well-being. The association asserts that retired men and women and other senior citizens have a right to live with dignity and security, to remain competent for most of their lives, and to serve as active participants in their communities. Inquiries from prospective members are encouraged at any time.

Publications: The ASCA publishes a bimonthly newsletter, *Senior Citizens Voice.*

American Society of   **ASCP**
Consultant Pharmacists
2300 9th Street, South
Arlington, VA 22204

(703) 920-8492

Profile: This national professional society of pharmacists provides pharmacy and consulting services to nursing homes, home health care facilities, and similar institutions and organizations. It maintains a directory of its members, some three thousand leading practitioners in the field. While the ASCP is not a consumer organization, it is in a position to make referrals for individuals desiring more information about prescription drugs and pharmaceutical products for patients in nursing homes and other extended-care facilities.

Publications: The ASCP publishes, in addition to its directory, a professional journal.

American Society of   **ASTA**
Travel Agents
1101 King Street
Alexandria, VA 22314

(703) 739-2782

Profile: The ASTA is a trade association representing more than twenty-one thousand travel agents in 129 countries. The association follows current developments in the travel industry and is active in setting standards to improve the industry. Through various communications programs, including a speakers' bureau, it informs the general public about tips for travelers, travel scams and frauds, the advantages of using a travel agent, and ways to pack more efficiently. The ASTA also supplies information for retirees, other older people, and the handicapped about tours that have special considerations for these travelers.

Publications: The ASTA distributes, or suggests, literature and books on all forms of travel, domestic and foreign.

American Society on Aging   ASA
Suite 512
833 Market Street
San Francisco, CA 94103

(415) 882-2910

Profile: The more than eight thousand members who make up the American Society on Aging serve as a strong force working for the well-being of elders, responding to today's needs and anticipating those of the future. The membership includes representatives of the public and private sectors, service providers, researchers, educators, advocates, health and social service professionals, and retired people. The ASA serves, too, as a clearinghouse for information on retirement and aging, provides information to the public about legislation that affects older people, and informs health professionals about available research programs. The ASA hosts some twenty conferences each year on aging and makes reports available for those interested.

Communications: The ASA publishes a bimonthly newspaper, *Aging Today,* and distributes booklets and audiovisual materials on aging, health care, senior housing, long- and short-term care resources, government programs for older people, retirement, and many other subjects.

American Speech-Language-Hearing Association   ASHA
10801 Rockville Pike
Rockville, MD 20852

(301) 897-5700

Profile: The ASHA is the national professional, scientific, and accrediting organization for more than sixty thousand speech-language pathologists and audiologists who treat speech, language, and hearing disorders. As the central source of information about such disorders, it communicates to the public through spokespersons, reports, and publications. Of particular concern to older people are speech disorders and hearing loss that come from aging or serious illnesses such as a stroke.

Communications: Literature is available on these disorders, preventive measures, and treatment through the association and its members.

American Tinnitus Association   ATA
PO Box 5
Portland, OR 97207

(503) 248-9985

Profile: The ATA is a voluntary organization whose basic objective is to support research to find a cure for tinnitus, constant buzzing or ringing noises in the ears or head, which occurs most often in people in their late fifties or older. The association sponsors self-help groups nationwide and offers information and support for tinnitus patients and their families. It also conducts continuing education programs for health professionals on the management of the disorder.

Publications: The ATA publishes a quarterly journal for members and other professionals and makes available a number of booklets for older readers, including *Information about Tinnitus* and *Coping with the Stress of Tinnitus.*

American Wheelchair   **AWBA**
Bowling Association
Larkspur Lane
Menomonee Falls, WI 53051

(414) 781-6876

Profile: The American Wheelchair Bowling Association was formed by a group of bowling enthusiasts who were confined to wheelchairs but wanted to continue the sport, both for enjoyment and exercise. The association has established special rules for handicapped participants, organizes and promotes wheelchair bowling leagues, and sponsors wheelchair bowling tournaments. It encourages inquiries from disabled people interested in bowling and provides information about the sport and where participation is available.

Amtrak Distribution Center
PO Box 2717
Itasca, IL 60143

(800) 368-8725

Profile: A department of Amtrak was formed to assist older people who want to travel by train but have problems because of age, infirmity, or disability. Retirees and other older people are also offered special discounts for rail travel, up to 25 percent. Inquiries are encouraged.

Amyotrophic Lateral Sclerosis   **ALSA**
(ALS) Association
15300 Ventura Boulevard
Sherman Oaks, CA 91403

(818) 990-2151

Profile: The ALSA was formed to provide funding for research and to distribute information about amyotrophic lateral sclerosis (ALS), commonly referred to as Lou Gehrig's Disease. The ALSA not only compiles all known data about this mysterious degenerative illness but also serves as a strong communicant to victims and their families while ALS runs its course. The association provides patients and specialists with the latest research data concerning the disease and treatments (many experimental) that have been developed.

Communications: The ALSA provides materials to help ALS patients live with the disease and the disorders associated with it and informs family members about methods for helping patients and themselves cope with the associated problems.

Andrus Gerontology Center   **AGC**
University of Southern California
University Park
Los Angeles, CA 90089-0191

(213) 743-5156

Profile: The Andrus Gerontology Center carries out a wide variety of research and educational activities through its Research Institute and the Leonard Davis School of Gerontology. As such, it is a major source of information for professionals and the public alike on the subject of aging. Of special interest is the center's course on retirement planning, which covers such subjects as: the physical, psychological, and social changes that occur in mid and later life; the impact of these changes on decision making and behavior; financial matters; physical and mental health; the use of leisure time; and resources for better retirement.

Communications: Older people and those preparing for retirement can obtain further information by contacting the center.

Arthritis Foundation   **AF**
PO Box 19000
Atlanta, GA 30326

(404) 872-7100
(800) 283-7800

Profile: The Arthritis Foundation funds and supports programs to find a cure for all (more than one hundred) forms of arthritis and regularly distributes information to professionals and the public on its findings. Local AF chapters, listed in the phone book, offer information and referral services to people with arthritis who are seeking help. The foundation also sponsors education programs for afflicted individuals, such as the Arthritis Self-Help Course, the Aquatic Program, and the Exercise Program.

Publications: The Arthritis Foundation publishes and distributes more than eighty booklets on the various types of arthritis, coping with the disease, the effects of various drugs and treatments, self-help tips, and many other related topics.

Asociacion Nacional   **ANPPM**
Pro Personas Mayores
Suite 270
2727 West Sixth Street
Los Angeles, CA 90057

(213) 487-1922

Profile: Founded in 1975, the ANPPM is a national membership organization committed to promoting coalitions nationwide to improve the well-being of older Hispanics and other low-income elderly. It conducts research about Hispanics and aging, produces and disseminates bilingual information and audiovisuals, provides training and technical assistance, and administers a nationwide employment program for low-income older persons.

Communications: Audiovisuals and publications on topics related to older Hispanics are available.

Associated Services for the Blind   **ASB**
919 Walnut Street
Philadelphia, PA 19107

(215) 627-0600

Profile: Associated Services for the Blind is a nonprofit organization providing the skills, tools, and resources for the independence of blind persons. Programs include retirement planning for the blind and visually impaired, rehabilitation, peer counseling, advocacy, and other social services. The ASB communicates through conventional media, braille, large-print publications, recordings, a speakers' program, and a closed-circuit radio station.

Communications: Older people who are blind or visually impaired and their families can contact the ASB for the types of materials described above.

Association for   ABTR
Brain Tumor Research
6232 North Pulaski Road
Chicago, IL 60646

(312) 286-5571

Profile: The ABTR is a voluntary organization committed to brain tumor research and to promoting better understanding of this disease and related disorders. The association funds researchers in medical centers around the country who are studying new methods of diagnosing and treating brain tumors, both benign and malignant. Association members offer information and moral support to patients with tumors and their families, and also suggest ways for establishing self-help groups.

Publications: The ABTR distributes a number of pertinent booklets to the public, including *A Primer of Brain Tumors* and *Coping with a Brain Tumor.*

Association for Continuing Higher Education   ACHE
c/o Executive Vice President
College of Graduate and Continuing Studies
Evansville University
Box 329
Evansville, IN 47702

(812) 479-2471

Profile: The ACHE was founded as a center for promoting interest in college-level continuing adult education on both a full-time and part-time basis. The association maintains a directory of adult education courses, particularly ones of interest to retirees and other elders, and can recommend further sources of information about specific types of institutions and subjects.

Publications: The ACHE distributes literature about programs, as well as source directories.

**Association for the Education
and Rehabilitation of the Blind
and Visually Impaired**
206 North Washington Street
Alexandria, VA 22314

(703) 548-1884

Profile: This association is committed to studying and implementing ways of rehabilitating people who are blind or visually impaired and helping them return to more normal patterns of living. It encourages inquiries from retired people who have suddenly had to face severe eyesight problems, and helps them to locate specialists and services and to cope with continuing low-vision problems.

Publications: The association publishes a monthly periodical devoted to jobs available to people with vision problems, and distributes pertinent literature and information upon request.

Association of Private Pension   **APPWP**
and Welfare Plans
Suite 1250
1212 New York Avenue, NW
Washington, DC 20005

(202) 289-6700

Profile: The APPWP represents a broad range of American companies, banks, insurers, and other allied professionals on retirement income, health care, and employee benefit issues. Association members are actively involved in matters involving retirees and older people, such as health care costs, health care services in retirement, expanding pension plans, personal taxation, age discrimination, and investments. The APPWP encourages inquiries from retirees and would-be retirees about these subjects, the availability of pertinent information, and prospects for the future.

Publications: The association makes available literature, fact sheets, and editorials on pension and welfare plans and related subjects.

Asthma and Allergy   **AAFA**
Foundation of America
Suite 305
1717 Massachusetts Avenue, NW
Washington, DC 20036

(202) 265-0265

Profile: The AAFA was founded to acquire and disseminate accurate information about asthma and other allergies and support ongoing research in this field. The foundation undertakes studies, educates professionals, and administers a continuing public relations program to inform people about disorders in this field. It offers assistance to retirees who move to new locations where they unexpectedly suffer allergy problems, and to older people in general who are afflicted with chronic allergic diseases.

Communications: The AAFA produces or distributes information and publications on all forms of allergic problems, including asthma, hay fever, skin disorders, and allergic reactions to foods, drugs, pollen, and insect bites.

Atrium Center
Senior Living Communications
Suite 300
1515 North Federal Highway
Boca Raton, FL 33432

(407) 392-4550

Profile: The Atrium Center was established as a publisher of newsletters about retirement and aging by a gerontologist, Dr. David Demko. Dr. Demko authors a newspaper column on senior living, which counsels retirees and other elders. Readers are encouraged to write letters of comment and inquiry to the center.

Publications: The Atrium Center publishes a bimonthly newsletter, *Resources in Aging,* described by Dr. Demko as "a comprehensive resource file on aging and the aged." It reports on such topics as Alzheimer's disease, prostate enlargement, Medicaid, the rights of elder patients, women and aging, retirement income, and patient-doctor relationships. It is available upon subscription.

Automotive Consumer Action Program   **AUTOCAP**
8400 Westpark Drive
McLean, VA 22102

(703) 821-7144

Profile: This program was established by the National Automobile
Dealers Association (NADA) as a means of resolving third-party
disputes relating to the purchase or performance of automobiles.
Older people who are dissatisfied with their cars and who cannot
obtain satisfaction through the local dealer involved have
recourse through AUTOCAP.

Bankcard Holders of America   **BHA**
560 Herndon Parkway, Suite 120
Herndon, VA 22070

(800) 638-6407

Profile: The BHA is a service that provides credit card information and computerized data to professionals and consumers. It
solicits inquiries from consumers interested in obtaining information, about credit cards and various kinds of credit card services,
among other things.

BBB Auto Line
Suite 800
4200 Wilson Boulevard
Arlington, VA 22203

(703) 276-0100

Profile: Auto Line was established by the Better Business Bureau
as a third-party dispute resolution program for the following
makes of cars: AMC, Audi, General Motors and its divisions,

Honda, Jeep, Nissan, Peugeot, Porsche, Renault, Saab, and Volkswagen. Car buyers who are dissatisfied and cannot obtain satisfaction from their local dealer can contact the BBB Auto Line to make a complaint.

Benefits Media, Inc.   **BMI**
301 14th Avenue
North Nashville, TN 37203

(615) 329-5014

Profile: BMI is a management consulting firm established in 1969, which offers products and services to human resource professionals. Although this is a for-profit organization and charges for its services, it informs individuals about locations where BMI-generated material can be reviewed. For example, it distributes films on retirement planning to its clients for presentation to pre-retirement audiences.

Publications: BMI distributes two paperback books: *So You're Hanging It Up,* a preretirement guide for government workers by George Biles, and *Retirement Is . . . a Rainbow High,* by Carol Ann Gautier.

Better Hearing Institute   **BHI**
5021B Backlick Road
Annondale, VA 22003

(703) 642-0580
(800) EAR-WELL

Profile: The Better Hearing Institute is a nonprofit educational institution that implements national public information programs on hearing loss and available assistance—medical, surgical, hearing aid, and rehabilitative—for people with uncorrected hearing problems. BHI produces public-service messages for radio, television, and print media, many of which have featured celebrities who overcame hearing loss. Among them are Arnold Palmer, Bob Hope, Phyllis Diller, Nanette Fabray, and Art Carney. Older people with hearing problems are encouraged to write the institute or phone the toll-free hotline, the 800 number given above, for information.

Publications: The BHI publishes a monthly newsletter, *Communicator,* with highlights of activities in this field, and distributes a number of informative booklets, such as *Overcome Hearing Loss Now!, Nerve Deafness and You, Tinnitus, or Head Noises,* and *We Overcame Hearing Loss,* with personal comments from well-known people.

Better Sleep Council   **BSC**
333 Commerce Street
Alexandria, VA 22314

(202) 333-0700

Profile: The Better Sleep Council is a nonprofit organization that sponsors a national awareness campaign to inform the public of the importance of proper sleep habits and the way in which bedding affects one's life and rest. The council undertakes studies of sleep habits and reports its findings to health professionals and the general public. Special information is available for retirees who may have trouble sleeping after changing habitats and environments and older people with sleep-disturbing disabilities.

Publications: The council distributes a number of free booklets on sleep habits and bedding and suggests books that can help resolve sleep problems. One example is a book sponsored by the BSC, *How to Sleep Like a Baby,* by sleep specialist Dianne Hales, published by Ballantine Books in 1987.

Better Vision Institute   **BVI**
Suite 1310
1800 North Kent Street
Rosslyn, VA 22209

(703) 243-1508

Profile: The Better Vision Institute was funded by the Vision Council of America to serve as a source of information on eye health and vision care. Through public information channels and educational materials, the BVI encourages people to take better care of their eyes, stressing the fact that vision problems often go long undetected. The institute provides information in a variety of ways on age-related vision disorders and how they can be anticipated and treated, and helps older people locate specialists when they are not under a physician's care or have retired and moved to a new location.

Publications: The institute publishes a professional newsletter and a number of useful pamphlets including *Vision Problems of the Aging,* and *Vision Care,* and reports on glaucoma, cataracts, sunglasses, the proper care of eyeglasses, and other vision-related subjects.

Beverly Foundation
Suite 750
70 South Lake Avenue
Pasadena, CA 91101

(213) 684-1100

Profile: The Beverly Foundation was established as a research group committed to the health and well-being of older people and a developer of programs to provide opportunities for "creative aging." The foundation has designed and administered a range of community demonstration projects that focus on the physical, social, and economic needs of America's older population. It works, too, with other age-related organizations to provide informative materials for this age group, as well as for health professionals and community service agencies. Of particular interest to retired people is the foundation's program to effect better ways of financing long-term care.

Publications: Numerous materials are made available by the foundation for the asking, examples of which are the booklets *Engaging in Aging* and *Homesharing for Older Adults* and a video training program for nursing assistants.

Boating Safety   **USCG**
United States Coast Guard
Department of Transportation
Washington, DC 20593

(202) 267-0780
(800) 368-5647

Profile: The Boating Safety division was formed to help owners of small boats enjoy their sport with greater pleasure and safety and a firmer knowledge of maritime laws and regulations. The Coast Guard encourages older people who are owners or users of small craft of every kind to obtain and read materials on these subjects before venturing into the ocean, lakes, rivers, or other waters.

Publications: Numerous booklets and other publications are readily available, either free or at reasonable cost, on all facets of boating and water safety.

B'nai B'rith International   BBI
1640 Rhode Island Avenue, NW
Washington, DC 20036

(202) 857-6580

Profile: Founded in 1843, B'nai B'rith is the world's largest Jewish organization, supporting community action programs of many kinds and working to improve the living conditions of disadvantaged people. B'Nai B'rith supports the arts and sciences, fights discrimination, promotes interfaith dialogue, and maintains visitation programs for persons who are sick or shut in. Many of its programs are devoted to the elderly, caring for those who are not well and providing housing for those who need shelter. The Senior Housing Program constructs and maintains apartment houses for retirees and older adults throughout the United States.

Publications: International Jewish Monthly is distributed to members and other interested persons. Also available are publications on aging, housing for seniors, and volunteer services for older people.

Boat Owners Association   BOA
of the United States
880 South Pickett Street
Alexandria, VA 22304

(703) 823-9550

Profile: Members of the association are the owners of pleasure boats of all kinds, whether for fresh- or saltwater use. The purpose of the association is to serve as an advocate for favorable legislation, to promote boating safety, to develop boat-handling courses and workshops, and to increase the number and quality of boat basins, navigable waterways, and other areas in which small boats are operated.

Publications: The association publishes a newsletter and distributes literature on such subjects as boat handling, water safety, guides to waterways, navigation, and weather watching. It also lists full-length paperbacks and hardcover books on boating for pleasure and reference.

The Box Project
PO Box 435
Plainville, CT 06062

(203) 747-8182

Profile: The Box Project's goal is to alleviate poverty by locating and matching volunteers throughout the United States with individuals and families who need communication, material aid, and educational assistance to varying degrees. The program encourages understanding, trust, and cooperation among people of diverse economic and geographic backgrounds. There are six ongoing projects through which these goals are fulfilled: Supportive Relationships, Information/Newsletters, Home Visits/Advocacy, Education/Scholarship, Special Services, and Management and General. All provide opportunities to reach out and help people in need with a minimum of bureaucracy and a great deal of personal support.

Publications: The Box Project publishes a monthly newsletter on subjects of direct interest to participants, *A Program of Friendship, Material Aid, Information, and Action.*

Canadian Association   **CARP**
of Retired Persons
27 Queen Street, East
Toronto, Ontario M5C2M6, Canada

(416) 363-8748

Profile: The Canadian Association of Retired Persons functions
much as the American Association of Retired Persons, offering a
wide range of services, publications, and educational programs to
its members.

Cancer Information Service   **CIS**
National Institutes of Health
Office of Cancer Communications
9000 Rockville Pike
Bethesda, MD 20892

(301) 496-5830
(800) 422-6237

Profile: The CIS was established by the National Institutes of
Health as a clearinghouse for information about all forms of cancer, their diagnosis, treatment, and ongoing research. It maintains
an extensive library on cancer and related diseases. The CIS
responds to requests from patients and their families, as well as
medical and health professionals, for current information.

Publications: The Cancer Information Service publishes a list of
available literature on cancer and distributes booklets to consumers at no cost upon request.

Catholic Charities
1319 F Street, NW
Washington, DC 20004

(202) 639-8400

Profile: Catholic Charities is a nonprofit social service organization whose purpose is to offer a broad range of services to people
in need. It sponsors educational workshops and leadership training institutes, provides speakers on Medicare and other topics of
concern to seniors, and serves as an advocate for older people in
matters of housing, health, Social Security benefits, employment
opportunities, and welfare. The services for seniors offered by
this widespread organization include counseling, foster family
programs, homemaking, institutional care, health clinics, retirement planning, and emergency assistance.

Publications: Catholic Charities publishes its own periodical,
Charities USA, ten times a year, and distributes practical booklets
on a wide variety of social service subjects to anyone who
requests information.

Catholic Golden Age   **CGA**
400 Lackawanna Avenue
Scranton, PA 18503

(717) 342-3294
(800) 233-4697

Profile: The CGA unites its members behind issues of concern to
Catholics in matters such as human rights, world peace, the elimination of poverty, and the improvement of life. Its special program for senior citizens focuses on these issues in general and,
more specifically, on matters of health care, medical costs, retire-

ment, Social Security benefits, and housing for older people. It encourages members to communicate about these problems and participate in programs to help solve them.

Publications: The organization publishes *CGA World* and occasional reports on its activities and programs.

Cemetery Consumer Service Council   **CCSC**
PO Box 3574
Washington, DC 20007

(703) 379-6426

Profile: The Cemetery Consumer Service Council was established as a body that consumers could turn to in any disputes regarding interments and cemeteries in the United States. Older people who have questions about cemeteries and burial procedures can obtain information and assistance through the CCSC.

Center for Auto Safety   **CAS**
2001 S Street, NW
Washington, DC 20009

(202) 328-7700

Profile: The Center for Auto Safety answers questions about the safety of any model or make of automobile. The CAS also helps settle disputes relating to state or national "lemon" laws when consumers feel they have purchased a vehicle that does not live up to expectations or that has been misrepresented in advertising or promotion by an automobile dealer.

**Center for Chronic Disease Prevention   CCDPHP
and Health Promotion**
1500 Research Boulevard, MS5P
Rockville, MD 20850

(301) 251-5180

Profile: The center was founded as a nonprofit organization to conduct research in the field of chronic disease prevention and to present its findings to professionals and the public. The CCDPHP will provide older people with information about all kinds of chronic diseases and related health problems and will refer them to local specialists for treatment and advice.

Publications: The CCDPHP publishes regular reports and distributes pamphlets on chronic disease and health programs to the public.

Center for Consumer Health Education   CCHE
Reston, VA 22091

(703) 860-9090

Profile: The center was established as an advocate for individual responsibility for better health. Its basic objective is to educate the public about the necessity of using preventive medicine to avoid all kinds of physical disorders. It also teaches older people methods for self-care and ways to avoid exposure to major communicable diseases. Inquiries by the public are encouraged.

Publications: The CCHE distributes booklets at no cost on health education, self-help methods, and the nature of communicable diseases.

Center for Older Learners

See the Institute of Lifetime Learning, page 176.

Center for Science   CSPI
in the Public Interest
1501 16th Street, NW
Washington, DC 20036

(202) 332-9110

Profile: The CSPI is a voluntary, nonprofit organization whose members hold positions in the scientific world and are interested both in exchanging ideas among themselves and disseminating knowledge about science to the general public. The center encourages inquiries from individuals, such as retirees who are interested in science or are pursuing hobbies that are scientifically oriented.

Publications: The CSPI publishes scientific reports for its members and also distributes booklets to the public at no cost, upon request.

Center for Social Gerontology   CSG
Suite 204
117 North First Street
Ann Arbor, MI 48104

(313) 665-1126

Profile: The mission of the Center for Social Gerontology is to enhance the lifestyle and well-being of older people through its research, educational programs, and technical assistance to professionals in this field. The center sponsors seminars on issues that affect older people, such as health care, legal rights, housing, and trusteeship. The CSG has developed detailed programs on specific problems, such as one to improve the care and welfare of patients afflicted with Alzheimer's disease.

Publications: The CSG publishes a professional journal and also makes available to the public a series of booklets on issues relating to its field of service.

Center for the Study of Aging   **CSA**
706 Madison Avenue
Albany, NY 12208

(518) 465-6927

Profile: The Center for the Study of Aging was established as a nonprofit organization to promote research and training in the field of aging. The center sponsors educational programs on health and fitness for professionals and the public, and offers professional assistance to researchers in the field of gerontology. The CSA makes available consultation services to professionals involved with the development of community programs and services for older people. These activities include retirement planning, physical fitness programs, nutrition, housing, and day care.

Communications: The CSA conducts a regularly scheduled radio program and makes available to the public free information booklets on topics related to aging, retirement, housing, changing family relationships, and the creative use of leisure time.

Children of Aging Parents   **CAP**
2761 Trenton Road
Levittown, PA 19056

(215) 547-1070

Profile: Children of Aging Parents is a nonprofit, self-help group whose purpose is to provide support and distribute information to family members taking care of older relatives who are lonely, infirm, or disabled. CAP administers a number of public programs, including Instant Aging Workshops for community groups. CAP also sponsors similar programs for professionals and social workers in hospitals, nursing homes, and rehabilitation centers. Retirees are encouraged to contact Children of Aging Parents if they find themselves being cared for by younger family members.

Publications: CAP publishes a monthly newsletter, *Capsule,* and distributes publications on ways to start a self-help group. Brochures include *Caring for the Alzheimer's Disease Patient, As Your Parent Grows Older,* and *The Sandwich Generation: Adult Children of the Aging.*

Citizens Emergency Center   **CEC**
Room 4811
US Department of State
Washington, DC 20520

(202) 647-5225

Profile: The Citizens Emergency Center was established by the Department of State as a unit that Americans can contact when traveling abroad and faced with an emergency. Examples of such occasions might be losing a passport or other critical documents, having to fly home unexpectedly because of death or illness in the family, or being caught in the throes of a foreign uprising. Older people who travel are particularly advised to know the contacts they can make immediately and reliably in the case of emergencies.

Citizens for a Better Environment   **CBE**
407 South Dearborn Street
Chicago, IL 60605

(312) 939-1530

Profile: Citizens for a Better Environment is a nonprofit organization that was established by people concerned about air and water pollution and other factors that unfavorably affect the environment. Members are dedicated to reducing exposure to toxic substances in the air, water, or on land, and encourage other individuals and groups to take positive action in this respect. The CBE makes environmental studies, provides information to the public, and engages in civil suits and court actions to prevent endangering the environment.

Publications: The CBE maintains an environmental library and distributes fact sheets and booklets to the public.

Civil Rights Division
Department of Justice
Washington, DC 20530

(202) 633-3847

Profile: This division of the Department of Justice was established specifically to take all necessary actions to protect the rights of American citizens. It defends individuals against all forms of discrimination, whether because of age, sex, race, color, national origin, or creed. It informs the public about individual rights and encourages people to protest and take action whenever they feel that these rights have been violated. Branches are maintained in all states and most major cities of the United States and can be found in the telephone directory under the listing for the Department of Justice in the United States Government Offices section.

| **Clearinghouse on Disability Information** | **CDI** |

Room 3132, Switzer Building
400 Maryland Avenue, SW
Washington, DC 20202-2524

(202) 732-1723

Profile: The Clearinghouse on Disability Information was created by the Rehabilitation Act of 1973 to respond to inquiries and research and document information about facilities serving the handicapped. The clearinghouse responds to inquiries on a wide range of topics, including aging, all kinds of physical and mental handicaps, education in this field, funding, and legislation affecting handicapped people. Older people, or those with small incomes, may qualify for assistance based on factors in addition to their handicaps. Or they may be eligible for special service and nutrition programs, such as Meals-on-Wheels or food stamps.

Publications: The clearinghouse distributes numerous booklets on disabilities as well as a very useful handbook, *Pocket Guide to Federal Help for Individuals with Disabilities.*

Clearinghouse on the Handicapped
Room 3132, Switzer Building
330 C Street, SW
Washington, DC 20202

(202) 732-1241

See Clearinghouse on Disability Information, page 129, whose functions overlap with this agency.

Commission on Civil Rights   **CCR**
Suite 606
1121 Vermont Avenue, NW
Washington, DC 20425

(202) 376-8116
(800) 552-6843

Profile: The Commission on Civil Rights serves, among other things, as an agency to which older people can turn if they feel that their rights have been violated because of age—or for any other reason.

Commission on Legal Problems   **CLPE**
of the Elderly
American Bar Association
1800 M Street, NW
Washington, DC 20036

(202) 331-2297
(800) 621-6159

Profile: The Commission on Legal Problems of the Elderly is a component of the American Bar Association that was formed to focus on the legal problems of older Americans. The CLPE responds to inquiries from individuals about such problems and maintains a referral service to put people in touch with attorneys and others who can assist them at little or no cost.

Publications: The CLPE distributes booklets and fact sheets on all kinds of legal problems that affect older people in such matters as wills, trusts, finances, housing, medical care, lawsuits, and negligence.

Committee on Human Development   CHD
University of Chicago
5801 South Ellis Street
Chicago, IL 60637

Profile: The Committee on Human Development acquires funds and supports ongoing research on many subjects in its field, the most pertinent being its research on retirement. Older individuals who are interested can contact the committee for information about studies that might be of interest.

Publications: The committee publishes research reports and papers on retirement and aging, among others, some of which are available to individuals upon request.

Community Action for Legal Services   CALS
Food Law Project
335 Broadway
New York, NY 10013

(212) 431-7200

Profile: Community Action for Legal Services was established to assist people with low incomes who are in need of legal counsel or assistance. The Food Law Project provides older individuals with information about federal, state, and local food and nutrition programs. Most services are free.

Publications: CALS distributes reports and booklets on legal matters at no cost and also lists related legal publications that are available for a nominal charge.

Comprehensive Pain Center   **CPC**
Department of Neurological Surgery
University of Miami School of Medicine
PO Box 016960
Miami, FL 33101

(305) 547-6946

Profile: The Comprehensive Pain Center is a unit of the School of Medicine of the University of Miami and is devoted to various rehabilitation programs, especially those involving the back. The center responds to requests from individuals about disorders that cause chronic pain and will refer them to facilities and specialists in their areas.

Concern for Dying
250 West 57th Street
New York, NY 10107

(212) 246-6962

Profile: Concern for Dying is a group whose objective is to compile, study, and communicate information about death and dying, to ease the pain of survivors, and to provide more dignity to the dying patient.

Publications: Concern for Dying distributes information in this subject field, including a booklet on living wills, and also provides information about other available literature of interest to older people and their families.

Con Edison
4 Irving Place
New York, NY 10003

(800) 522-5635

Profile: Con Edison maintains an Enlightened Energy program for its utility customers in each region it serves, one objective of which is to inform users of electricity and gas about ways to improve air-conditioning and heating efficiency, conserve fuel, and save money. While the information the company provides is regional, the methods and approaches are ones that can be utilized almost nationwide. Con Edison encourages inquiries from individuals.

Publications: The company publishes *Concern Spotlight*, aimed at an audience of older people who have signed up for its "Concern" program, and distributes numerous free booklets, such as *Enlightened Energy*, on ways to save fuel and utility costs.

Consumer Alert   CA
Suite 425
1024 J Street
Modesto, CA 95354

(209) 524-1738
(202) 296-1148 (Washington, DC, office)

Profile: Consumer Alert is a nonprofit nationwide consumer organization with members in all fifty states. It promotes competitive enterprise, works to increase competition in the marketplace, and serves as a watchdog to detect practices that are harmful to consumers. Among its functions and actions are the economic analysis of consumer issues, exposing the hidden costs of government regulation, protecting the environment, disseminating data on automobile and highway safety, and studying the safety and nourishment of foods and food products.

Publications: Consumer Alert distributes releases and fact sheets on the above issues and others.

Consumer Information Center   **CIC**
PO Box 100
Pueblo, CO 81002

Also:
GSA Room G142
18th and F Streets, NW
Washington, DC 20405

(202) 501-1794

Profile: The Consumer Information Center is a unit of the General Services Administration (GSA), which was established in order to help government agencies provide the public with useful information on a wide spectrum of subjects. Many of the booklets and fact sheets are free; full-length books are available at varying costs.

Publications: The center publishes its *Consumer Information Catalog* four times a year, which lists more than two hundred government publications of interest to consumers. Many of the titles are of specific interest to older readers, covering such subjects as housing, retirement, benefits, insurance, nutrition, health, recreation, hobbies, crafts, and financial matters.

Consumer Product Safety Commission   **CPSC**
Washington, DC 20207

Also:
Room 332
5401 Westbard Avenue
Bethesda, MD 20207

(301) 492-6580
(800) 638-CPSC

Profile: The CPSC was formed by the federal government to effect safety standards that would protect consumers against injury from faulty products. This agency helps to evaluate the safety of all types of consumer products, promotes research related to the causes and prevention of product-related injuries, and warns the public about unsafe products that have reached the marketplace. The CPSC sets mandatory standards for manufacturers, monitors industry, and requires reports on product defects as soon as they are detected. The toll-free hotline, the 800 number given above, responds to inquiries from the public about products, equipment, and materials that are hazardous and could cause injury or illness.

Publications: The CPSC publishes a list of booklets that are available free to the public, such as *Home Safety Checklist for Older Consumers.*

Consumers Union of the United States   **CU**
256 Washington Street
Mount Vernon, NY 10553

(914) 667-9400

Profile: The Consumers Union is a widely recognized organization that was established to research, study, and test multitudes of consumer products and materials and provide information to the public. Many such reports compare competing brands in regard to performance, quality, and cost. The CU also serves as an advocate, representing consumer interests in the courts and in local and national legislation.

Publications: The CU publishes *Consumer Reports,* a monthly magazine available by subscription, a newsletter, and a wide variety of paperback and hardcover books at various prices on automobiles, appliances, food, insurance, and other subjects of interest to consumers.

Council for the Elderly   **CE**
1909 K Street, NW
Washington, DC 20036

(202) 662-4933

Profile: The Council for the Elderly is an affiliate of the American Association of Retired Persons (AARP), whose commitment is to providing legal service and counsel to older people at little or no cost in times of need. The council administers training programs to instruct attorneys and volunteer laypersons on ways to act as advocates on major issues affecting older people, including retirement benefits, legal rights, housing, health, insurance, trust funds, and death benefits. The council maintains an Outreach Program for older people who are shut-ins or confined to an institution.

Publications: Facts sheets and reports are available upon request, on related topics.

Council of Better Business Bureaus   **CBBB**
Consumer Information
4200 Wilson Boulevard
Arlington, VA 22203

(703) 276-0100

Profile: The Council of Better Business Bureaus is an organization that serves to coordinate the activities of Better Business Bureaus (BBBs) located across the United States. Its mission is to collect and distribute information to the public about all matters pertaining to the ethical and legal conduct of business and charitable organizations. The council, through its local affiliates, sponsors numerous public information programs; works closely with regulatory agencies at the federal, state, and local levels; and alerts itself to current and pending legislation regarding business practices and policies. Consumer inquiries and complaints are encouraged and should be directed to local Better Business Bureau offices. In recent years, the CBBB has increasingly pinpointed investigations into practices that concern older people and their well-being, covering such topics as fraudulent health schemes, mismanaged housing developments, and questionable investment programs.

Publications: The CBBB and its affiliates publish regular reports and newsletters on their activities, distribute free pamphlets on request, and sponsor full-length paperbacks and hardcover guidebooks on subjects of concern to consumers. One such book is *Investor Alert! How to Protect Your Money from Schemes, Scams, and Frauds,* by Wilbur Cross, published by Andrews and McMeel in 1988.

Council on Family Health   **CFH**
420 Lexington Avenue
New York, NY 10017

(212) 210-8836

Profile: The Council on Family Health is a membership organization for manufacturers of prescription drugs and medications that are sold over the counter. The CFH conducts studies and provides the professional community and the public with data about drugs and their proper and effective usage. One facet of this program relates to prescriptions and medications used by older people and the relationship of their effectiveness to the age of the user. The council investigates other aspects of family health, including home safety and procedures to follow in the case of medical emergencies.

Publications: Fact sheets, reports, and booklets are available through the CFH on many of the subjects described above.

Country Music Association   **CMA**
PO Box 22299
Nashville, TN 37202

(615) 244-2840

Profile: The Country Music Association was the first trade organization formed to promote a particular type of music and is made up of more than seven thousand music professionals. Claiming some one hundred million fans today, the CMA reports that a large percentage of these people are in their late fifties or older. The CMA communicates regularly with fans through radio, television, and print media, and hosts the CMA Awards Show, the International Country Music Fan Fair, and numerous professional growth seminars.

Communications: The CMA publishes newsletters and releases on its programs and responds readily to inquiries and requests from fans.

Credit Union National Association   CUNA
PO Box 431
Madison, WI 53701

(608) 231-4014

Profile: CUNA was established as a clearinghouse of information on financial planning, credit, money management, and related topics. It maintains a file of data of particular interest to retired people and other seniors. Upon request, it sends booklets, data sheets, and other printed matter on the above subjects to consumers.

Cross Country Ski Areas Association   CCSAA
259 Bolton Road
Winchester, NH 03470

(603) 239-4341

Profile: The Cross Country Ski Areas Association promotes skiing by providing information to the press and generating media coverage of cross-country skiing. The CCSAA disseminates information to the general public on safety, skiing etiquette, and how to get started in this sport. It also publishes information on ski areas and equipment and sponsors trade shows and regional meetings to inform professionals and the public about advances in cross-country skiing techniques and equipment. Some programs focus on this form of skiing as an appropriate form of exercise for older people who want to maintain their fitness but are not qualified to participate in downhill skiing.

Publications: These are restricted mainly to releases and professional bulletins, but the CCSAA responds to individual requests for information.

"Dear Abby"
Ms. Abigail Van Buren
PO Box 447
Mount Morris, IL 61054

Profile: Ms. Van Buren, who writes the "Dear Abby" column, offers publications from time to time on a variety of subjects relating to readers' welfare and activities. Older readers are advised to keep an eye out for such publications or to write her to inquire about subject areas of interest.

Delta Society
PO Box 1080
Renton, WA 98057-1080

(206) 226-7537

Profile: The Delta Society was formed as a voluntary, nonprofit association to study and administer programs that use animal pets as a form of therapy for older people and the handicapped. Branches of the society furnish trained cats, dogs, birds, and other pets to extended-care centers, nursing homes, hospitals, and hospices to improve the well-being of patients who are shut in or disabled. In some cases, pets are placed on loan with individuals who are qualified to care for them and who benefit from this form of companionship. The society works closely with local humane associations to locate suitable pets and recruits and trains volunteers to work with the institutions and individuals who are recipients. All veterinary care, including shots and medical attention, are provided by the Delta Society.

Publications: Delta publishes *Anthrozoos,* a quarterly that discusses the interactions of people and animals, and on request will provide a list of pet-therapy programs and the communities where they are available or planned.

Design for Aging
American Institute of Architects
1735 New York Avenue
Washington, DC 20006

(202) 626-7459

Profile: The Design for Aging program of the American Institute of Architects was created as a means of creating residences that are attractive yet at the same time functional for and compatible with older people. Designs incorporate such features as halls and corridors that are wide enough to accommodate wheelchairs, a minimum of steps, improved lighting, and fixtures that can be easily used by people with decreased hand and arm mobility. The AIA provides information to its members about Design for Aging features and responds to inquiries from older people about the availability of architects and designers who specialize in residences for older people.

Dial-a-Hearing Screening Test
Occupational Hearing Services
PO Box 1880
Media, PA 19063

(800) 222-3277
(800) 222-EARS
In Pennsylvania: (215) 565-6114

Profile: Phone calls to the above numbers will provide an individual with information on hearing problems and treatments. The service also provides information on the federal government service for the hard-of-hearing known as Telecommunication Device for the Deaf, or TDD. These devices enable people who have hearing and/or speech impairments to communicate via telephone by typing a message on the device's keyboard. (Many federal government offices now have TDD numbers, most of them in the 202 area code.)

Diet Workshop   **DW**
Suite 300
Hearthstone Plaza Building
111 Washington Street
Brookline, MA 02146

(617) 739-2222

Profile: Diet Workshop is a mutual self-help organization for people who are overweight. It takes the stand that overeating can be reduced by generating peer support among members. To this end, older members and retired people form subgroups to support one another. The workshop studies and recommends certain kinds of food products and provides information on diets that are healthy, nutritious, and low in calories.

Direct Mail Marketing Association   **DMMA**
6 East 43rd Street
New York, NY 10017

(212) 689-4977

Profile: The DMMA was established by individuals and organizations in the direct mail industry to establish ethical standards, study marketing methods, and coordinate functions with related groups. The DMMA responds to inquiries from consumers about mailing systems and practices, and hears complaints about such matters as "junk mail" and literature promoting questionable products and services.

Publications: The DMMA produces manuals, data books, and fact sheets on direct mail subjects.

Direct Selling Association   **DSA**
1776 K Street, NW
Washington, DC 20006

(202) 293-5760

Profile: The Direct Selling Association is composed of members who are in the business of direct sales or related functions. The mission of the DSA is to improve the image of direct ("door-to-door") selling, establish standards of procedure and conduct, and weed out fly-by-night firms that have in the past given this field of salesmanship a bad name. Through print and broadcast media, releases, and other communications, the association communicates the benefits of making direct purchases. People can also obtain information about direct selling opportunities in their areas by contacting the DSA.

Publications: The DSA publishes newsletters and reports on direct selling activities and maintains lists of firms that seek retirees and other consumers to act as sales representatives.

Disabled American Veterans   **DAV**
807 Maine Avenue, SW
Washington, DC 20024

(202) 554-3501

Profile: The DAV is a private, nonprofit organization that represents veterans of American wars who have service-connected wounds, injuries, or other disabilities. The DAV helps these veterans to obtain housing, jobs, and free or low-cost health care; assists in filing claims for Veteran's Administration (VA) benefits or disability compensation; and looks into such matters as pensions and death benefits. The Older Veteran Assistance Program is specially designed to aid senior men and women who have service-related disabilities and provide support for their families.

Publications: The association publishes *DAV Magazine* monthly and periodically distributes materials on issues of concern to older veterans. Lists of free publications are available from the DAV service offices located in each state.

Displaced Homemakers Network   **DHN**
1010 Vermont Avenue, NW
Washington, DC 20005

(202) 628-6767

Profile: Founded in 1979, the DHN addresses the specific concerns of women who have been homemakers for years but have abruptly lost financial support because of death, divorce, separation, or disability. The network's objectives are to assist displaced homemakers in becoming financially independent, to provide information about public policy issues, to provide technical assistance for service providers, and to help professional participants in the DHN apply their knowledge to the improvement of programs. More than nine hundred local programs offer individual counseling and supportive services, often to older women who have few relatives to turn to for help.

Publications: The DHN publishes *Network News* quarterly, as well as numerous free pamphlets that address the problems of displaced homemakers. A list of these publications is available upon request.

Elder Health Program
School of Pharmacy
University of Maryland
20 North Pine Street
Baltimore, MD 21201

Profile: The Elder Health Program is a university-sponsored research and study project, which sponsors educational programs in the field of health and medicine, with emphasis on older people and medications. People with problems concerning prescription drugs or other medications can obtain referrals to sources of information by writing directly to the program.

Elderhostel
Suite 400
80 Boylston Street
Boston, MA 02116

(617) 426-8056

Profile: Elderhostel consists of a network of more than 1,500 colleges, universities, culture centers, museums, and other educational institutions that offer low-cost, short-term residential academic programs for people who are sixty and older. Programs are offered throughout the United States and Canada and in more than forty countries overseas, the domestic ones averaging one week in length and those abroad lasting two or three weeks. Elderhostel provides an informal and compatible atmosphere where the individual is important, making friends is easy, and the effects of the educational programs are stimulating. Costs are moderate. A fee of about $250, for example, covers most courses in the United States for one week, including room and board, tuition, all classes, the use of campus recreational facilities, and a variety of extracurricular activities.

Publications: The Elderhostel *Catalog,* a tabloid-size publication, is updated quarterly and is free upon request.

Employee Benefit Research Institute   **EBRI**
2121 K Street, NW
Washington, DC 20037

(202) 659-0670

Profile: The Employee Benefit Research Institute is a private, nonprofit, nonpartisan public-policy research organization. Through research, policy forums, workshops, and educational publications, the EBRI contributes to the dissemination of knowledge in the field of public and private employee benefit plans, and to the formulation of effective retirement planning programs devoted to health and welfare after retirement.

Publications: The EBRI publishes reports and fact sheets and provides printed information on such subjects as retirement planning, pensions, and continuing benefits.

Entrepreneur magazine
2392 Morse Avenue
Irvine, CA 92714-9440

(800) 421-2300

Profile: _Entrepreneur_ is the major magazine that promotes start-ing and maintaining one's own business. Published monthly, it provides case histories of entrepreneurs who have been success-ful in fields ranging from auto repairing and bookselling to innkeeping, printing, showmanship, and yogurt making. During the course of a year, the magazine reviews just about every kind of franchise imaginable and publishes an annual directory of some one thousand franchises, with statistics about the type of ownership, start-up cost, royalties, financing, advertising, and profitability. Since many franchises and small, entrepreneurial businesses are launched by retirees, this leading magazine in its field is a must for older people considering such ventures.

Publications: In addition to its monthly magazine and special issues, the publisher of _Entrepreneur_ produces fact sheets and literature on various kinds of franchises and entrepreneurial ventures.

Environmental Action   **EA**
1525 New Hampshire Avenue, NW
Washington, DC 20036

(202) 745-4870

Profile: Founded by the organizers of the first Earth Day, EA is a nonprofit organization whose members undertake environmental research projects, lobby for covering legislation, and engage in public education and grass-roots assistance. EA's areas of special-ization include air quality, energy efficiency, toxic materials, global warming, and waste reduction. EA encourages inquiries and solicits volunteers from older people concerned about the state of our planet.

Publications: EA publishes reports and releases on subjects concerning the environment, pollution, and ecology.

Environmental Protection Agency   **EPA**
Public Information Center
401 M Street, SW
Washington, DC 20460

(202) 382-2080

Profile: The EPA is the federal government agency that is responsible for controlling pollution and protecting the environment. Its programs set standards for maintaining the land, air, and water and providing safe drinking water throughout the United States. Individuals who want to report problems or have inquiries are encouraged to contact the EPA or its affiliated agencies that protect us against such pollutants as pesticides, asbestos, and toxic waste.

Publications: The EPA distributes numerous booklets to the general public, including *Asbestos in the Home, Safe Drinking Water,* and *A Citizen's Guide to Radon.*

Epilepsy Foundation of America   **EFA**
4351 Garden City Drive
Landover, MD 20785

(301) 459-3700

Profile: The EFA was established to foster research in the field of epilepsy and related brain disorders and seizures, seek better methods of treatment for patients, and provide support for epileptics and their families. The foundation sponsors educational programs and seminars for professionals in medicine and health and serves as a clearinghouse of information for them and the general public as well. The foundation responds to inquiries from laypersons and refers them to local resources for further information and assistance.

Publications: The EFA publishes professional journals and papers on epilepsy and distributes leaflets and fact sheets to individuals upon request.

Eye Bank Association of America   **EBAA**
Suite 308
1725 Eye Street, NW
Washington, DC 20006-2403

(202) 775-4999

Profile: Each year, some forty thousand people in North America have their sight restored by corneal transplant surgery through the services of the Eye Bank Association of America. The EBAA is a nonprofit organization that maintains about one hundred eye banks located across the nation. It also supports research in this field, maintains educational programs for professionals, and provides the general public with information.

Publications: Information on eye transplants and related subjects can be obtained by contacting the EBAA.

Facts on File
460 Park Avenue South
New York, NY 10016

(800) 322-8755

Profile: Facts on File is a for-profit publishing organization that produces factual books on a wide variety of topics for distribution to libraries, other public institutions, health and welfare groups, and the general public. Its catalog includes fifty or more books, for example, on medicine, covering such topics as aging, environmental hazards, alcoholism, later-life health, nursing homes, respiratory and infectious disorders, heart disease, diabetes and digestive ailments, insomnia, headaches, and physical fitness, diet, and nutrition programs. For a catalog of individual reference books, contact Facts on File at the address above or use their free phone number.

Families United   **FUSAF**
for Senior Action Foundation
1334 G Street, NW
Washington, DC 20005

(202) 628-3030

Profile: The Families USA Foundation is a nonprofit organization committed to maintaining the well-being and security of older Americans and their families. Its focus is on providing better services and specialists in the fields of home care, long-term care, health programs, economic security, Medicare, Social Security, and productive and creative opportunities for seniors. The FUSAF supports studies in these fields, sponsors programs to educate professionals, and communicates with the general public on matters of common interest.

Communications: The foundation distributes printed matter and audiovisuals on subjects of interest to older people and their families.

Family Motor Coach Association   **FMCA**
8291 Clough Street
Cincinnati, OH 45244

(513) 474-3622

Profile: The members of the Family Motor Coach Association are owners of self-propelled, self-contained motor homes and coaches who are interested in exchanging ideas and information, acting as advocates of legislation beneficial to their mode of travel, and desirous of planning recreational camp-outs and rallies. The FMCA studies and sponsors highway safety programs, examines and reports on new types of vehicles and equipment, and promotes better public understanding and recognition. The association responds to inquiries from retirees and other seniors interested in joining the FMCA or learning more about motor homes and coaches.

Family Service America   **FSA**
Park Place
11700 West Lake Park Drive
Milwaukee, WI 53224

(414) 359-2111

Profile: The mission of Family Service America is to study, evaluate, and publish information about activities, events, and programs in the human services field. The subject areas with which the FSA has recently become involved include retirement, legislation on behalf of the elderly, marital therapy, family public policy, crisis intervention, substance abuse, financial management, the concerns of older women, and living with stress. The FSA supports and sponsors programs for National Family Week, held annually each fall, and invites inquiries about its areas of involvement.

Publications: The FSA publishes a journal, *Families in Society,* as well as books on the above-mentioned and related subjects. It also produces audio and videotapes, including a fourteen-program video course on health care for professional use. A catalog will be sent upon request.

Family Service Association of   **FSA**
Nassau County, Inc.
336 Fulton Avenue
Hempstead, NY 11550

(516) 292-2600

Profile: Typical of family assistance organizations across the country, this association is a multiservice human services agency that serves a variety of purposes relating to older people and their families. Among its programs for senior citizens are Project SHARE, a shared housing program; CHEC, a counseling program for seniors interested in home equity conversions; LINK-AGE, a broad-based program that links seniors to a wide range of services; and Senior Financial Counseling, which offers retirement planning, estate management, tax advice, and debt counseling.

Publications: The association publishes brochures on shared housing, home equity, finances, domestic problems, aging, and many other topics, and also suggests other sources of information.

Family Support Administration   **FSA**
370 L'Enfant Promenade, SW
Washington, DC 20447

(202) 252-4796

See United States Department of Health and Human Services, page 292.

Federal Council on the Aging   **FCA**
Room 4545
330 Independence Avenue, SW
Washington, DC 20201

(202) 245-2451

Profile: The FCA is an advisory group authorized by the Older Americans Act of 1965, whose fifteen members are selected by the president and the Congress to represent a cross-section of rural and urban older Americans and national organizations with an interest in aging, business, labor, and the general public. The council reviews and evaluates federal policies and programs that affect retirees and older Americans, and makes recommendations to Congress, the president, the Department of Health and Human Services, and the commissioner on aging. The council also conducts or commissions research on aging and sponsors seminars to discuss the problems and needs of older people.

Publications: The council publishes an *Annual Report* and distributes data on aging.

Federal Crime Insurance Program   **FCIP**
PO Box 6301
Rockville, MD 20850

(800) 638-8780

Profile: The Federal Crime Insurance Program was established to study the impact of crime on the nature and cost of all forms of insurance affected by criminal acts and activities. The FCIP refers inquiries to local agencies that can provide specific data on crime insurance. This kind of information can be useful to people planning retirement and looking for areas that are relatively crime free.

Federal Deposit Insurance Corporation   **FDIC**
550 17th Street NW
Washington, DC 20429

(202) 389-4221
(800) 424-5488

Profile: The FDIC monitors complaints against federally insured banks that are not members of the Federal Reserve System. It communicates with the public through various media and handles consumer complaints about alleged violations of fair-credit provisions. Older people are encouraged to contact a regional office of the FDIC, which can be reached through the toll-free 800 number above, if they have questions or complaints.

Publications: The FDIC publishes and distributes literature of interest to consumers, including *Equal Credit Opportunity and Age, Fair Credit Billing, Truth in Lending,* and *Your Insured Deposit.*

Federal Home Loan Bank Board   **FHLBB**
Office of Thrift Supervision
1700 G Street, NW
Washington, DC 20552

(202) 906-6237
(800) 842-6929

Profile: The Federal Home Loan Bank Board was established to answer questions from consumers about the Federal Home Loan Bank System, the Federal Savings and Loan Insurance Corporation, and the Federal Home Loan Mortgage Association, among other things. The board makes studies and investigations in these areas and dispenses information to professionals and the general public.

Publications: The FHLBB distributes free publications on its activities and subjects related to the institutions named above.

Federal Information Centers   **FIC**
26 Federal Plaza
New York, NY

(212) 264-4464

Profile: Federal Information Centers are located in major cities in thirty-six states, listed under "Federal Information Center" in the phone book. These centers were established to help individuals find information about federal government services, programs, and regulations. FICs can also tell you which government agency to contact for help with problems.

Federal Trade Commission   **FTC**
Office of Public Affairs
Room 421
6th Street and Pennsylvania Avenue, NW
Washington, DC 20580

(202) 523-3598

Profile: The FTC is the federal government agency that establishes trade regulations and protects consumers from unfair or
deceptive business practices. It maintains ten regional offices, in
addition to the Washington, DC, headquarters. FTC consumer
protection programs relate to the fair packaging and labeling of
products, truth in advertising, product reliability, fair credit
reporting, direct-mail advertising, door-to-door sales, and the
business practices of nursing homes and other facilities for the
elderly.

Publications: The FTC distributes free literature on subjects with
which it is involved, including services for older people, advertising practices, credit, franchises and business opportunities, and
investment fraud.

Federation of Fly Fishing   **FFF**
PO Box 1088
West Yellowstone, MT 59785

(406) 646-9451

Profile: Members of this association are aficionados of serious
sport fishing, many of whom tie their own flies. Retirees interested in becoming members or learning more about sports fishing techniques and equipment are invited to inquire.

Fifty-Plus Runners Association
PO Box D
Stanford, CA 94305

(415) 723-9790

Profile: This association is composed of older men and women who have found running to be their most desirable way to health and physical fitness. The association promotes competition, holds meets, and provides guidelines for senior runners and those interested in taking up the sport.

Publications: The association publishes a newsletter and distributes informational pamphlets on running as a beneficial form of exercise.

Food and Nutrition Information Center   **FNIC**
Room 304
National Agricultural Library Building
Beltsville, MD 20705

(301) 344-3719

Profile: The role of the Food and Nutrition Information Center is to provide information to professionals and the general public on foods, nutrition, food services, and food technology. The library maintains an extensive collection of books, audiovisual materials, recordings, and technical papers. A special section is devoted to nutrition for retired people and the elderly in need of special diets. The library is open to the public on weekdays from 8:00 A.M. to 4:30 P.M., EST.

Publications: Bibliographies and resource guides are available on diets, nutrition, dental health, vegetarianism, and diet and health for older people, as well as material on the relationship between nutrition and the prevention of certain diseases.

Food Safety and Inspection Service   **FSIS**
Department of Agriculture
14th Street and Independence Avenue, SW
Washington, DC 20250

(202) 447-7943

Profile: The FSIS was established as a service to maintain research files and inform the public about ways of preventing food and drink contamination. To this end, the FSIS sponsors public-service advertising campaigns and other communications services to reach professionals and the public. A special program is devoted to food contamination problems that are particularly hazardous for older people.

Publications: The FSIS distributes free pamphlets on the prevention of food contamination and ways to detect whether foods and drinks are safe.

Footwear Council   **FC**
51 East 42nd Street
New York, NY 10017

(212) 581-7737

Profile: The Footwear Council is one of several organizations devoted to the history, design, manufacturing, and marketing of shoes, boots, slippers, and related products. The council has made special studies on the footwear needs of older people and can supply literature and referrals for consumers who wish to obtain further information. The council can also suggest associations of foot specialists who care for the feet and ankles and are qualified to make recommendations.

Ford Consumer Appeals Board
PO Box 1805
Dearborn, MI 48126

(313) 337-6950
(800) 241-8450

Profile: The Ford Consumer Appeals Board was established to receive and act on complaints from consumers about new cars that turned out to be "lemons" or about other problems relating to Ford vehicles.

Foster Grandparent Program   **FGP**
The Federal Domestic Volunteer Agency
1100 Vermont Avenue, NW
Washington, DC 20525

(202) 634-9108

Profile: Since 1965, foster grandparents and children with special needs have formed a winning combination. Most foster grandparents are retired or low-income seniors who receive a modest hourly stipend for their service, though some with modest incomes do serve without any payment. Foster grandparents attend to the physical, mental, and emotional needs of disadvantaged children, acting as caring individuals who provide stability to a child's world. Foster grandparents also do volunteer work in schools for the mentally retarded, in Head Start programs, and in juvenile detention centers. Retirees and other older people interested in this form of service are urged to contact Foster Grandparent programs in their areas or get in touch with ACTION (see page 48) for further information.

Foundation for Grandparenting   **FG**
Box 31
Lake Placid, NY 12946

Profile: The Foundation for Grandparenting is a nonprofit organization dedicated to the betterment of society through intergenerational involvement. Since 1980, it has been involved in conceiving and implementing grandparent/grandchild programs and projects nationally and internationally. Older people who serve as grandparents work with individual youngsters or in programs that take place in schools, camps, day care centers, and wherever children are gathered in groups for education, recreation, or other activities.

Publications: The Foundation for Grandparenting publishes *Vital Connections: The Grandparenting Newsletter,* which contains case histories and stories about grandparenting. A sample copy can be obtained by sending a stamped, self-addressed envelope to the above address.

Foundation for Hospice   **FHH**
and Homecare
519 C Street, NE
Washington, DC 20002

(202) 547-7424

Profile: The Foundation for Hospice and Homecare is composed of community agencies providing homemaker home health services, through which individuals are cared for in their own homes by qualified professionals. Working with other health and welfare agencies, the FHH works to effect a better understanding of home health services for older people who are seriously or terminally ill. The foundation provides support, establishes standards

and procedures, conducts educational seminars, administers programs, and solicits funds and volunteers to assist professionals.
Individuals are encouraged to contact the foundation either to
volunteer services or to seek help.

Publications: The FHH publishes *HomeCare News* biweekly,
along with several other periodicals, and distributes consumer literature such as *All about Homecare, Family Caregiver's Guide,*
and *Consumer's Guide to Hospice Care.*

Foundation for Infectious Diseases
Box 42022
Washington, DC 20015

*See National Institute of Allergy and Infectious Diseases, page
230.*

Garden Club of America   GCA
598 Madison Avenue
New York, NY 10022

(212) 753-8287

Profile: The Garden Club of America was founded by amateur
gardeners interested in exchanging ideas about the growing of
flowers and decorative plants and making studies to determine
better ways of pursuing their hobby or avocation. The GCA
sponsors educational programs, promotes flower and garden
shows, hosts garden tours, and distributes books and brochures
on all aspects of the subject. Inquiries are invited from retirees
who would like to become members or are seeking further
information.

Gerontological Society of America   **GSA**
Suite 350
1275 K Street, NW
Washington, DC 20005-4006

(202) 842-1275

Profile: Founded in 1945, the GSA is a membership organization of professionals whose role is to study and promote the development and dissemination of knowledge about aging. The GSA is a society involved with research, practice, and education, and is structured around four basic disciplines: biological sciences; clinical medicine; behavioral and social sciences; and social research, planning, and practice. Older people are encouraged to contact the society for information about aging.

Publications: The GSA produces a number of professional and technical papers and distributes consumer information to the public.

Glaucoma Foundation   **GF**
310 East 14th Street
New York, NY 10003

(212) 260-1000

Profile: The Glaucoma Foundation was established to undertake research and communicate information about glaucoma, one of the most common and least understood of all diseases and the second leading cause of blindness in the United States. The foundation sponsors research, conducts seminars, and informs the public through major media about this widespread eye disease, which can strike all ages but is particularly prevalent in older people. Those with questions or inquiries are encouraged to contact the GF for information or referrals to specialists in their areas.

Publications: The Glaucoma Foundation publishes professional papers and reports, but also distributes consumer leaflets, such as *About Glaucoma,* to the general public.

Golden Age Passports   **GAP**
National Park Service
US Department of the Interior
18th and C Streets, NW
Washington, DC 20240

(202) 343-4747

Profile: The Golden Age Passports division of the National Park Service was established to provide helpful information to older people about facilities and tours in America's national parks. It provides counsel on special facilities for older people who are infirm or handicapped and makes available special discounts for seniors.

Golden Companions
PO Box 754
Pullman, WA 99163

(509) 334-9351

Profile: Golden Companions is a travel companion network and newsletter exclusively for people who are fifty or older. Members come from all walks of life and all regions of the United States, as well as from Canada, Mexico, and abroad. The common goal of members is to find traveling companions by referring to confidential biographies that describe members but identify them only by code number. Confidentiality is retained for as long as each member desires. Golden Companions organizes group tours to many parts of the world. Membership, $60, entitles members to confidential exchange information, a bimonthly newsletter, discounts from national tour agencies, a vacation home exchange listing, social get-togethers, and Golden Companion tours and cruises.

Publications: Golden Companions publishes releases, informational literature, and a newsletter, *The Golden Traveler.*

Golden Pen Pal Association   GPPA
of North America
1304 Hedgelawn Way
Raleigh, NC 27615

Profile: The GPPA is composed of older men and women, in many cases those who are shut-ins or physically disabled, who want to correspond with their peers. Although the association is basically North American, the correspondence of members is by no means limited to this continent and, indeed, has spread to many countries abroad.

Grandparents Association of America   GAA
PO Box 2410
Peachtree City, GA 30269

(404) 455-1616

Profile: The GAA was formed by older people interested in developing communications and relationships with grandchildren and other young people whom they "adopt" as grandsons or granddaughters. The GAA also serves as an advocate to sponsor and support legislation favorable to seniors.

Publications: The association publishes a newsletter and distributes occasional literature on the relationships between older adults and young people.

Grandparent's/Children's Rights   GCR
5728 Bayonne Avenue
Haslett, MI 48840

(517) 339-8663

Profile: Founded in 1981 and now having affiliated groups in some forty states, the GCR is composed of grandparents and other older men and women dedicated to protecting the rights of children, especially those who are emotionally, mentally, physically, or sexually abused. One of the GCR's basic objectives is to lobby for federal, state, and local laws to safeguard the rights of children and protect the visitation rights of grandparents. The GCR serves as a clearinghouse for information on these subjects and will provide data or make referrals to people who phone or write.

Gray Panthers
Suite 601
311 South Juniper Street
Philadelphia, PA 19107

(215) 545-6555

Profile: The motto of the Gray Panthers is Age and Youth in Action. From the beginning, the membership has been open to persons of all ages and concerned with issues affecting all ages. One of the major goals is to educate the public about the negative affect of ageism, or age-based discrimination, in our society. Local chapters organize groups of young and older people to work together to develop better health care, transportation, housing, and employment opportunities for older individuals. The organization also works to effect legislation that will fight discrimination and improve the welfare of older people. Through its Margaret Mahler Institute, the association awards grants to researchers and

creative artists over the age of seventy who need financial assistance to continue to lead dignified and useful lives.

Publications: The Network Newspaper is distributed quarterly to
members and subscribers. Posters and publications on subjects of
interest to members are available free or at low cost.

Green Thumb
5111 Leesburg Place
Falls Church, VA 22041

(703) 820-4990

Profile: Green Thumb was established as an organization to help
provide job training and find full- or part-time employment for
older men and women, particularly seniors living in rural areas of
the United States. Inquiries are invited from people who fit this
category.

Guide Dog Foundation for the Blind   **GDFB**
171 East Jericho Turnpike
Smithtown, NY 11787

(516) 265-2121

Profile: The GDFB was established as a means of training dogs to
lead the blind and matching them with compatible owners whom
they can lead safely in the course of daily life, even across busy
streets. It is estimated that about 10 percent of the blind population can use these animals successfully. The foundation conducts
research, schedules indocrination sessions (generally about a
month for the blind person, after the dog itself has been trained),
and acquaints the public with its ongoing programs. Information
and literature are available, as well as referrals and references to
full-length books.

Leonard J. Hansen
P.O. Box 90279
1326 Garnet Avenue
San Diego, CA 92169-0279

(619) 272-7262

Profile: Leonard J. Hansen authors a weekly newspaper column, *Mainly for Seniors,* published through Copley News Service and running in 230 daily and weekly newspapers around the nation. He is also the author of *Life Begins at 50: A Handbook for Creative Retirement Planning.* This large-size, 352-page paperback is published by the Avery Publishing Group and available in bookstores for $11.95. Hansen will respond to requests from seniors about retirement. Send him a stamped, self-addressed envelope at the above address.

Headache Research Foundation   **HRF**
Faulkner Hospital
Allandale at Center Street
Jamaica Plain, MA 02130

(617) 522-7900

Profile: The HRF was established primarily to make studies and conduct research on headaches, their types, causes, treatments, and cures. The organization serves as a clearinghouse of data for medical and health professionals, patients, and their families. A basic role of the foundation is to communicate with the public, as well as with the professionals, and emphasize the fact that headaches are often serious disorders or symptoms of serious diseases. The HRF provides free information, refers inquirers to local sources of information and assistance, and sponsors educational programs for professionals and laypersons.

Publications: In addition to professional papers, the foundation distributes booklets on the various types of headaches, causes, self-help procedures, and treatments.

Health Care Financing Administration   **HCFA**
US Department of Health and Human Services
Suite 658
East High Rise Building
6325 Security Boulevard
Baltimore, MD 21207

(202) 245-6145
(800) 638-6833

Profile: Created in 1977, the HCFA has oversight of the Medicare and Medicaid programs and related medical care quality-control staffs. It also sponsors health care quality-assurance programs, such as the Second Surgical Opinion Hotline, the 800 number listed above. The HCFA establishes eligibility requirements for health care recipients, prepares claims procedures for health care providers, and coordinates activities between professionals and laypersons.

Publications: In addition to professional journals, the HCFA distributes booklets of interest to consumers, such as *Thinking of Having Surgery?* and *Guide to Health Insurance for People with Medicare.*

Health Information Center   **HIC**
PO Box 1133
Washington, DC 20013

(800) 336-4797

Profile: The HIC was established as a clearinghouse for information on health research, care, and facilities. The center provides referral service for older people who want to obtain specific data on health care subjects.

Health Resources   **HRSA**
and Services Administration
5600 Fishers Lane
Rockville, MD 20857

(301) 443-2086

Profile: The HRSA was established to study and evaluate health services of many kinds that are available to the general public. It acts as a clearinghouse of information for professionals and laypersons and refers inquirers to specific sources of data.

Healthcare Abroad
Suite 923, Investment Building
1511 K Street, NW
Washington, DC 20005

(202) 393-5500

Profile: This agency was established as a source of information about health care for people traveling outside the United States. It provides information and counsel for older Americans who have health problems and need to know in advance what facilities and types of specialists they can expect to find in the countries and regions they intend to visit.

Heart Life
PO Box 54305
Atlanta, GA 30308

(404) 523-0826
(800) 241-6993

Profile: Heart Life is a private, nonprofit organization dedicated to supporting heart patients and their families. It provides background information, makes referrals, and helps individuals and organizations establish local self-help groups. Inquiries are invited.

Helen Keller National Center   **HKNC**
111 Middle Neck Road
Sands Point, NY 11050

(516) 944-8900

Profile: This national center was established in honor of the late Helen Keller who, though blind and deaf herself, devised many ingenious ways of living a very full life without sight or hearing. The mission of the center is to circulate information about blindness to the public, support research to prevent and treat visual impairment in every degree, sponsor educational programs, and counsel the blind on ways in which to overcome their disadvantage.

Publications: The center distributes information about blindness and the use of aids to help the visually impaired, and it refers inquirers to the many articles and books that have been written by and about Helen Keller.

High Blood Pressure Information Center   **HBPIC**
120-180 National Institutes of Health
Bethesda, MD 20892

(301) 951-3260

Profile: The HBPIC was established as a branch of the National Institutes of Health to serve as a clearinghouse for data on high blood pressure, its causes, symptoms, and treatment. The center provides referral services for patients and their families seeking further information, specialists, or facilities for treatment.

Publications: The center publishes fact sheets and releases on high blood pressure and distributes free booklets about the disease, upon request.

Hillhaven Foundation
1148 Broadway
Tacoma, WA 98401-2264

(206) 572-4901

Profile: Hillhaven Foundation sponsors research, educational programs, national conferences, and community forums in the fields of long-term care, geriatrics, and gerontology. It provides educational materials for professionals and information for the public on topics of concern to older people, and responds to inquiries about aging and health care.

Publications: The foundation publishes professional reports and releases and distributes booklets of interest to older people.

Hospice Association of America   **HAA**
519 C Street, NE
Washington, DC 20002

(202) 547-6586

For information on Hospice programs through HAA, see the list-
ing for its parent organization, National Association for Home
Care, page 195. Ask for free brochures on Hospice.

Household International   **HI**
2700 Sanders Road
Prospect Heights, IL 60070

(708) 564-5000

Publications: Through its parent company, Money Management
Institute, HI publishes a complete Money Management Library
of thirty-two-page brochures on subjects relating to personal
finance, many of them of particular interest to retirees. Among
the titles are *Your Retirement Dollar, Your Savings and Invest-*
ment Dollar, Your Insurance Dollar, Your Housing Dollar, Your
Food Dollar, Managing Your Credit, and *Your Financial Plan.*
Individual books cost $1.25 each and the complete library of
twelve books, with a slipcase, is $12.00.

Human Nutrition Information Service   **HNIS**

See the United States Department of Agriculture, page 292.

Huntington's Disease   **HDSA**
Society of America
250 West 50th Street
New York, NY 10107

(212) 757-0443
(800) 345-4372

Profile: The mission of the HDSA, a voluntary, nonprofit organization, is to sponsor research about Huntington's disease, a hereditary, degenerative neurological disorder, and to support and serve patients suffering from it. The society, through its hotline, the 800 number given above, offers crisis intervention, genetic counseling, and referral services weekdays from 9:00 A.M. to 5:00 P.M., EST. The HDSA also sponsors self-help groups around the country for individuals with Huntington's disease and their families.

Publications: The organization publishes *The Marker,* a quarterly magazine, as well as consumer booklets on home care, research, development, and other pertinent topics.

Information for the Partially Sighted
9012 Old Georgetown Road
Bethesda, MD 20814

(301) 493-6300

Profile: This organization is an information resource that counsels people who are not blind but visually impaired. It studies and recommends assistive devices and helps patients qualify for large-print library books, recordings, and other services at little or no cost.

Institute for Aerobics Research   IAR
12330 Preston Road
Dallas, TX 75230

(214) 701-8001
(800) 527-0362

Profile: The mission of the IAR is to study and evaluate aerobics, a system of vigorous physical exercise, sometimes combined with dance routines, designed to stimulate the circulation of blood and heighten breathing. The institute, which has conducted studies on the value of aerobics for people who are sixty and older, provides information on request and will also make referrals to local sources of information and available programs.

Institute for the Hispanic Elderly   IHE
105 East 22nd Street
New York, NY 10010

(212) 677-4181

Outside of the New York City area, see the Asociacion Nacional Pro Personas Mayores, page 109.

Institute of Aging   IA
University of South Florida
4202 East Fowler Street
Tampa, FL 33620

Profile: The Institute of Aging is a private, nonprofit organization supported by the University of South Florida whose purpose is to conduct studies and undertake research on the process of aging. Though most of the institute's findings are directed at physicians and other health professionals, referrals are made for laypersons who inquire or request publications.

Institute of Certified   **ICFP**
Financial Planners
Suite 320
Two Denver Highlands
10065 East Harvard Avenue
Denver, CO 80231

(303) 751-7600

Profile: The ICFP is an association of professionals whose members are concerned with developing standards of ethical conduct and procedure, providing service to consumers, and disseminating information about the role of financial planning in the matter of investments and other personal economic programs. The ICFP maintains a code of ethics, supports full disclosure of the background and experience of financial planners, and reviews complaints and conflict-of-interest disputes. It also holds continuing educational seminars for professionals and financial-planning orientations for consumers.

Publications: The ICFP publishes a quarterly *Journal of Financial Planning* and a bimonthly newsletter, *Institute Today,* that present digests of issues affecting the profession and the public.

Institute of Gerontology
University of Florida
Gainesville, FL 32611

Profile: The Institute of Gerontology is a private, nonprofit organization supported by the University of Florida whose purpose is to conduct studies and undertake research on the process of aging. Though most of the institute's findings are directed at physicians and other health professionals, referrals are made for persons who inquire or request publications.

Institute of Lifetime Learning   **ILL**
1909 K Street NW
Washington, DC 20049

(202) 872-4700

Profile: The Institute of Lifetime Learning was founded in 1963
as a pioneer in learning projects for older people and is now a
clearinghouse of educational programs for seniors. It also provides technical assistance to institutions, disseminates information
to the public, develops new opportunities for older learners, and
seeks to enhance existing ones. Retirees who are interested in
furthering their education or acquiring knowledge about certain
subjects for any purpose are encouraged to contact the institute.

Publications: The institute publishes numerous brochures and
booklets, for both educators and laypersons, including *College
Centers for Older Learners,* descriptions of programs, and a
Directory of Centers for Older Learners, which covers this field
state by state.

Insurance Information Institute   **III**
110 William Street
New York, NY 10038

(212) 669-9200

Profile: The Insurance Information Institute was founded by the
insurance industry as a clearinghouse for information about
insurance policies and coverage of all kinds. It can provide background information and specific details on policies involving
such matters as health, long-term care, dentistry, hospitalization,
retirement plans, and other forms of coverage of special interest
to older people. The institute can also recommend sources of

information and assistance to people who feel that they have been discriminated against in being denied coverage or having claims rejected.

Publications: The institute distributes free booklets on many insurance topics upon request.

International Association for	**IAMAT**

International Association for   **IAMAT**
Medical Assistance to Travelers
417 Center Street
Lewiston, NY 14092

(716) 754-4883

Profile: IAMAT was established by physicians and others in the medical profession as an aid to travelers abroad, and particularly to those with chronic disorders or disabilities requiring regular care and not-infrequent emergency treatment. The association publishes a regularly updated directory of English-speaking doctors in some 500 cities in 120 countries. Contact the IAMAT for details and allied services.

International Association   **IAWP**
for Widowed People
PO Box 3564
Springfield, IL 62708

Profile: The mission of the IAWP is to provide a support group for widows and widowers, many of whom are recently bereaved and overcome with a sense of loneliness or depression, or unable to function as they had before. Members help each other during initial periods of grief and join in various programs sponsored by the IAWP, which include travel plans and services, group projects, the setting of realistic goals, social gatherings, and in some instances assistance in locating employment or meaningful volunteer jobs.

Publications: The IAWP publishes a directory of its membership and programs and distributes a number of booklets of interest to older people who have become widowed.

International Association   **IAG**
of Gerontology
Box 2948
Duke University
Durham, NC 27710

(919) 684-3416

Profile: The IAG is a private, nonprofit organization supported by Duke University's School of Medicine. Its mission is to conduct studies and undertake research in the field of gerontology on an international scale. Although most of the association's studies are for the benefit of medical specialists and other health professionals, referrals are made for the benefit of persons who inquire or request publications.

International Executive   **IESC**
Service Corps
PO Box 10005
8 Stamford Forum
Stamford, CT 06904-2005

(203) 967-6000

Profile: The IESC is an organization whose members are largely retired executives who volunteer to assist entrepreneurs who are starting their own businesses or may be having managerial problems with their business ventures.

International Federation on Aging   **IFA**
1909 K Street, NW
Washington, DC 20049

(202) 662-4987

Profile: The IFA is an international, nonprofit federation whose function is to conduct studies on aging worldwide in conjunction with major regional organizations, such as the United Nations, UNESCO, and the Council of Europe, and publish papers and books on their findings. These studies cover such subject areas as home-help services for older people, the process of aging in small native villages, mandatory retirement (blessing or curse?), crimes against the elderly, the status of older women in world social structures, and the advantages and disadvantages of shared living.

Publications: The federation publishes a free catalog of available books and other works, with descriptions and prices.

International Society for   **ISFRP**
Retirement Planning
11312 Old Club Road
Rockville, MD 20852-4537

(301) 881-4113
(800) 327-ISRP

Profile: The major objective of the ISFRP is to study many aspects of growing older and outline procedures to help people who are planning their retirement years. Such plans include all facets of retirement living, such as housing, health, social life, security, continuing education, nutrition, transportation, finances, investments, and relationships with dependents and other family members. The ISFRP responds to inquiries, provides basic information, and makes referrals to sources of specific data.

Interstate Commerce Commission   **ICC**
Office of Consumer Assistance
Constitution Avenue and 12th Street, NW
Washington, DC 20423

(202) 275-7844

Profile: The ICC is the agency of the federal government that regulates interstate transportation. Among other things, the ICC provides supervision and protection in the use of commercial moving companies to transport household goods and materials across state borders, as in the case of retiring to a new home. Older people who are planning a long-distance move can obtain useful booklets from the ICC that provide all the information they need on selecting the right mover, packing, and unpacking. The ICC is also an agency to fall back on in the event that claims or disputes arise between mover and customer that cannot be resolved at the local level. The ICC invites inquiries.

Investment Company Institute   **ICI**
1600 M Street, NW
Washington, DC 20036

(202) 293-7700

Publications: The ICI distributes a number of free booklets that are helpful to retired people trying to make wise investments to protect their savings and make their capital grow. One example is *A Translation: Turning Investment-ese into Investment Ease.* The brochure interprets the jargon of the investment world in clear language and provides helpful tips on lining up investment goals and priorities.

Jewish Association for   JASA
Services for the Aged
40 West 68th Street
New York, NY 10023

(212) 724-3200

Profile: The JASA was established to assist elderly people of the Jewish faith to remain in their communities if they so desire and to learn about the various agencies and services that are available to meet their needs. The JASA makes studies, conducts adult education programs, provides help for shut-ins, and in some cases allocates financial aid in time of need. The JASA also distributes a number of free publications on aging, housing, health care, and retirement.

Kellogg Foundation
400 North Avenue
Battle Creek, MI 49016

(616) 968-1611

Profile: The Kellogg Foundation is a philanthropic institution established in 1930 by W. K. Kellogg. Its interests have steadily broadened to include the support of projects throughout the world, with a focus on the application of knowledge in the fields of agriculture, education, and health. Recent studies have focused on the relationship between health and aging.

Legal Services for the Elderly   **LSE**
132 West 43rd Street
New York, NY 10036

(212) 391-0120

Profile: The LSE is an advisory center whose members are primarily attorneys specializing in the legal problems of older persons. The LSE does not provide services directly to clients but rather offers advice, memoranda of law, and briefs to other attorneys who serve older clients.

Publications: The LSE makes available a number of publications for the general public, including A *Survey of Legal Problems of the Elderly, Mandatory Retirement,* and *Savings for Seniors.*

Legal Research and Services   **LRSE**
for the Elderly
925 15th Street, NW
Washington, DC 20005

(202) 347-8800

See Legal Services for the Elderly, above.

Leukemia Society of America   **LSA**
733 Third Avenue
New York, NY 10017

(212) 573-8484

Profile: The Leukemia Society of America obtains funds and supports research to find a cure for leukemia and other diseases of blood-forming tissues. Through local chapters, it provides financial assistance to needy patients and helps to form support groups for patients and family members.

Publications: The LSA publishes a bimonthly newsletter, which reports on the society's activities and research. A list of informative booklets for consumers is available on request.

LifeSpan Communications, Inc.   **LCI**
51 East 90th Street
New York, NY 10128

(212) 678-0913

Profile: LifeSpan Communications is a private New York research firm that examines the impact of the mass media on the fifty-plus market. Its products and services include promotions, programs, direct marketing, public relations, marketing research, and strategic planning for both short- and long-range objectives. According to LCI, people who are fifty and older account for 47 percent of the audience for prime-time TV, 46 percent of daytime TV watchers, 37 percent of newspaper readers, and 33 percent of magazine readers. The company offers consultation on marketing, among other services, for retirees who own and manage their own businesses and want to know more about prospective clients and buyers who are in the older age bracket.

Lifeplan
Metropolitan Community College
3200 Broadway
Kansas City, MO 64111

(816) 756-0220

Profile: Lifeplan is a community education program that focuses on the medical, social, psychological, and financial aspects of aging. It provides preretirement training to individuals through public and group-sponsored seminars, preparing individuals and their families for the inevitable changes in lifestyle that occur when a person retires. Seminars are presented by health professionals, physicians, attorneys, accountants, and trained volunteers, thus allowing Lifeplan to present a flexible, comprehensive program for about $50 per participant. For further information, contact the office listed above.

Literacy Volunteers of America   LVA
700 East Water Street
Syracuse, NY 13210

(315) 445-8000

Profile: The LVA trains groups and individuals to serve as volunteers tutoring adults in basic reading or conversational English. The organization provides instructional materials and conducts workshops. This kind of program is duplicated by similar projects throughout the United States.

Little Brothers-Friends   LBFE
of the Elderly
National Headquarters
1121 South Clinton Street
Chicago, IL 60607-4416

(312) 786-0501

Profile: With "Flowers before Bread" as its motto, the LBFE is part of an expanding international, nonsectarian human-service organization that originated in France and was chartered in the United States in 1959. Composed largely of volunteers, many of whom are themselves older, it is dedicated to serving the lonely and isolated elderly throughout the world. Affiliates are located in Boston, Chicago, Minneapolis/St. Paul, Philadelphia, San Francisco, and the Upper Peninsula of Michigan. Interested retirees are encouraged to contact one of the regional offices or the headquarters listed above.

Lungline, National Asthma Center

(303) 355-5864
(800) 222-5864

Profile: This is a hotline, run by the National Asthma Center, for patients with asthma who have emergency situations regarding their breathing and need instant help or advice.

Lupus Foundation of America   LFA
Suite 203
1717 Massachusetts Avenue, NW
Washington, DC 20036

(800) 558-0121

Profile: The Lupus Foundation is a patient-oriented organization that conducts research and works to promote public awareness of this chronic inflammatory disease and develop better ways to diagnose and treat it. Local chapters of the LFA, listed in the phone directory, provide emotional support, encouragement, and help to patients and their families.

Publications: The foundation publishes *Lupus News* quarterly and a list of informative publications that are available on request.

Magazine Publishers of America   **MPA**
575 Lexington Avenue
New York, NY 10022

(212) 752-0055

Profile: The MPA, the industry association for consumer magazines, is committed, among other things, to establishing standards
for advertising and promotion and for improving the image of
magazines among other media in the eyes of the consumer. In
this respect, the MPA serves as a useful contact when readers
have unresolved complaints about subscriptions, feel that advertising is misleading or fraudulent, or take issue with the contents
or viewpoints of magazines.

Mail Order Action Line   **MOAL**
Direct Mail Association
6 East 43rd Street
New York, NY 10017

(212) 689-4977

Profile: People who are deluged with "junk mail" and want to get
off some of their mailing lists can solve the problem, at least in
part, by contacting MOAL. The organization cannot help with all
mailings, but can be of service in regard to any members who
belong to the Direct Mail Association.

Major Appliance   **MACAP**
Consumer Action Panel
20 North Wacker Drive
Chicago, IL 60606

(312) 984-5858
(800) 621-0477

Profile: MACAP is committed to helping consumers achieve fair resolution of complaints about major appliances that cannot be resolved through contacts with the local dealer or service agency, appliance manufacturer, or brand name retailer. The scope of products reviewed by MACAP includes washers and dryers, dishwashers, refrigerators, ranges, food waste disposers, dehumidifiers, freezers, microwave ovens, room air conditioners, and trash compactors. For information or to report complaints, contact the panel at the above address, local phone number, or 800 hotline.

Mature Outlook
6001 North Clark Street
Chicago, IL 60660-9977

(800) 336-6330

Profile: Formerly the National Association of Mature People, Mature Outlook is a paid membership organization for seniors that offers a great many benefits and services. These include, among others, medical and health programs; home, auto, and other insurance policies; travel and vacation planning; savings on eye examinations, eyeglasses, and other vision products; car rental discounts and highway emergency assistance; and worldwide discounts at restaurants, hotels, motels, and other facilities. Call the toll-free 800 number above for membership rates and literature describing the organization and its benefits.

Publications: The organization publishes *Mature Outlook,* a monthly consumer magazine for seniors, and distributes a variety of booklets, discount coupons, and fact sheets to members.

Meals-on-Wheels

For an address and phone number, consult "Department of the Aging" in your local telephone directory, under state, county, or municipal listings.

Profile: Meals-on-Wheels is a nonprofit service, staffed largely by volunteers, that delivers hot meals to older people who are shut in, especially those who have low incomes and no one at home to help.

MedEscort International
A-B-E Airport
Box 8766
Allentown, PA 18105

(215) 791-3111

Profile: MedEscort International is a group of medical professionals who are specially trained travel companions for the elderly or the handicapped. Services include travel coordination and transportation services worldwide by commercial air carriers and private medically equipped aircraft. MedEscort provides a door-to-door service by accompanying clients from origin to destination point, making all the necessary arrangements, including pretrip preparation and anything that needs to be accomplished prior to departure, such as errands, obtaining passports, or packing.

Publications: MedEscort publishes a booklet about its services and can also help inquirers to obtain travel literature of all kinds.

Medic Alert Foundation International
Turlock, CA 95381-1009

(209) 668-3333
(800) 344-3226
(800) ID-ALERT

Profile: Medic Alert is a nonprofit charitable organization that encourages individuals who are older or have health problems to carry identification and descriptions of their medical condition. Although there is a one-time fee of $25 for all services, people with low incomes are enrolled without charge at the request of a physician. The identification (ID) system is especially critical for persons with medical problems that are not readily apparent, such as epilepsy, diabetes, or allergies. The ID system consists of a bracelet or necklace worn by the patient, a wallet card containing updated data about the individual's health condition, and a twenty-four-hour answering service, which can be phoned collect by emergency personnel anywhere in the world.

Publications: Medic Alert publishes leaflets describing its services, such as *This Is Medic Alert, Medic Alert Response Service, Implant Registry,* and *Links to Life,* as well as releases and fact sheets.

Medicare
Department of Health and Human Services
Health Care Financing Administration
6325 Security Boulevard
Baltimore, MD 21207

(800) 638-6833
Hotline: (800) 344-3226

Profile: Medicare is the government health insurance program available to people who are sixty-five and older. It pays a large proportion of health care expenses but it does not pay them all. Participants face restrictions on some covered medical services, supplies, and equipment and must assume certain costs called deductibles and co-payments. Coverage includes doctors and outpatient services, some prescription drugs, hospital costs, skilled nursing facility care, and clinical examinations. However, the Medicare program is quite complicated, works in coordination with medical insurance plans, and is constantly changing. People in the Medicare program or about to qualify for it are advised to consult with medical authorities currently familiar with the system.

Publications: Numerous Medicare leaflets and fact sheets are available upon request, published by private insurance companies as well as by the federal government.

Mended Hearts   **MH**
7320 Greenville Avenue
Dallas, TX 75231

(214) 750-5442

Profile: Mended Hearts is a supportive organization composed of members who have successfully undergone major heart surgery. Local groups provide information to patients contemplating heart surgery and to their families. Older people with heart problems are encouraged to contact Mended Hearts for information about the organization and local contacts they can make.

Publications: Some groups publish informal newsletters and/or fact sheets, and most have on file photocopies of newspaper and magazine articles that have been published on Mended Hearts and members who are alive and active today because of the heart surgery they underwent in the past.

Money Management Institute   **MMI**
2700 Sanders Road
Prospect Heights, IL 60070

(708) 564-5000

See the entry for Household International and its Money Management Library, page 172.

Mountain States Health Corporation   **MSHC**
PO Box 6756
1303 Fort Street
Boise, ID 83707

(208) 342-4666

Profile: The MSHC is a private corporation serving retired people and the elderly in the Mountain States region of the United States. It makes studies, sponsors public-education programs, and will respond to older people who have questions about health resources and procedures.

National Academy of   **NAELA**
Elder Law Attorneys
Suite 108
655 North Alvernon Way
Tucson, AZ 85711

Profile: The National Academy of Elder Law Attorneys is a voluntary, nonprofit organization composed of lawyers and others in
the legal profession who specialize in handling legal problems for
retired people and the elderly. It undertakes studies to determine
the special legal needs of older people in all matters such as housing, wills, trusts, health plans, and discrimination. It responds to
inquiries at no cost and makes referrals to attorneys and legal services qualified to handle individual problems at little or no cost.

Publications: The NAELA distributes fact sheets and releases on
legal problems of the elderly and what they can do about them.

National AIDS   **NAIC**
Information Clearinghouse
PO Box 6003
Mail Stop 1B
Rockville, MD 20850

(800) 458-5231

Profile: The NAIC receives funds from the Centers for Disease
Control (CDC) to provide information and counsel to medicine
and health professionals about AIDS education programs and
services. It maintains the 800 hotline listed above for inquiries
from the public on weekdays from 9:00 A.M. to 7:00 P.M., EST,
and answers questions about the disease, prevention, treatment,
and the location of medical services.

Publications: The NAIC distributes free booklets, reports, and fact sheets on the disease, such as *Coping with AIDS* and *The AIDS Patient at Home.*

**National Alliance of   NASC
Senior Citizens**
2525 Wilson Boulevard
Arlington, VA 22201

(703) 528-4380

Profile: The role of the NASC is to serve as a consumer group to advocate policies and practices that improve the welfare of older people. It provides information to health professionals and the general public about retirement, health, housing, and the special needs of senior citizens, and lobbies federal and state governments for legislation on these issues. Benefits made accessible for members of the alliance include discounts on prescription drugs, health insurance, eye-care products, car rentals, and travel accommodations and meals. The alliance also has a program to establish retirement residences and life-care centers.

Publications: The NASC publishes two magazines, *Senior Guardian* monthly and *Our Age* bimonthly.

National Amputee Golf Association   NAGA
PO Box 1228
Amherst, NH 03031

(603) 673-1135

Profile: The members of the NAGA are largely golfers who love to play the game and are determined to do so despite the fact that they have lost an arm or a leg or are otherwise disabled. Other members are people whose avocation or profession is assisting the disabled. The association also encourages the physical, mental, and emotional rehabilitation of amputees through learning and playing golf, and it organizes golf programs and tournaments for these people.

Publications: The NAGA publishes a newsletter and distributes literature about golf as a beneficial sport for the disabled.

National Arthritis   NAIC
Information Clearinghouse
Box AMS
Bethesda, MD 20892

(301) 496-0211

Profile: The clearinghouse is a service of the National Institutes of Health to assist health professionals and the public in the location of current data about arthritis, musculoskeletal disorders, and skin diseases. It provides references for a federal computerized index that includes data on many diseases, health programs, and treatment centers, and produces reports and audiovisual materials for training programs.

Publications: The clearinghouse publishes a list of available materials free to the public, including bibliographies and fact sheets about arthritis and related diseases.

National Association for   NAHS
Hearing and Speech
10801 Rockville Pike
Rockville, MD 20852

(301) 897-8682
(800) 638-8255

Profile: The NAHS was established as a voluntary, nonprofit organization to educate the public about speech and hearing impairments and courses of action that can be taken to treat and minimize the problems. The association makes studies, underwrites research, and serves as an advocate of legislation to assist people with such impairments. A special focus is on the problems of the elderly. The NAHS responds to inquirers and refers them to local services where they can obtain advice and assistance.

Publications: The association publishes professional papers and also a directory of institutions in the United States that have devices to assist people with hearing impairments.

National Association for   NAHC
Home Care
519 C Street, NE
Washington, DC 20002

(202) 547-7424

Profile: The mission of the NAHC is to represent a variety of agencies that provide home care services, including home health agencies, hospice programs, and homemaker/home health aid groups. The association helps to develop proper professional standards and codes of ethics for agencies providing such care, sponsors continuing education programs for health professionals, and monitors federal and state legislation that affects older people and home care services.

Publications: The NAHC publishes several professional periodicals and distributes free publications on home care to consumers.

National Association for	**NASLI**
Senior Living Industries	
125 Cathedral Street	
Annapolis, MD 21401	
(301) 263-0991	
(301) 858-5001	

Profile: The NASLI is a private, nonprofit resource network of organizations, professionals, and individual citizens concerned with the quality of life for America's older population. The association makes studies, conducts research, and sponsors seminars on the special needs and problems of retired people and the elderly. It serves, too, as an advocate for legislation beneficial to older people. The NASLI encourages inquiries from older people and makes referrals to sources of further information and help.

Publications: The NASLI publishes a newsletter and professional papers and distributes consumer literature on aging and related subjects.

National Association for   NASSE
Spanish Speaking Elderly
Suite 219
2025 I Street, NW
Washington, DC 20006

(202) 293-9329

Profile: Like the Asociacion Nacional Pro Personas Mayores (page 109), the NASSE works to ensure that older Spanish-speaking citizens are included in all social-service programs for Americans in their age group. The association studies the needs of elderly Hispanics, serves as an advocate in initiating and enforcing legislation beneficial to them, and organizes programs to find employment for people fifty-five and older. It also serves as a catalyst in starting volunteer groups to serve low-income seniors. The NASSE encourages inquiries from the elderly and maintains bilingual answering and referral services.

Publications: The association publishes a regular bulletin and provides articles and booklets in Spanish on such topics as retirement, health, housing, Social Security, Medicare, and legal matters.

National Association for the Deaf   NAD
814 Thayer Avenue
Silver Spring, MD 20910

(301) 587-1788

Profile: The National Association for the Deaf is a volunteer, nonprofit organization which circulates facts about deafness and the problems of people with impaired hearing. It acts as a clearinghouse for information, lobbies for better legislation on behalf of the deaf, supports studies and research, and promotes the use of devices to aid the deaf in public places. NAD makes referrals for inquirers who need assistance and makes available its complete listing of organizations throughout the United States that provide services to the deaf and their families.

Publications: NAD publishes two magazines, *The Deaf American* quarterly and *Broadcaster* monthly, and distributes books and other printed materials on deafness and sign language. A catalog of publications is available at no cost upon request.

National Association for   NAHE
the Hispanic Elderly
2727 West Sixth Street
Los Angeles, CA 90057

(213) 487-1922

See the Asociacion Nacional Pro Personas Mayores, page 109.

National Association of   NAILC
Independent Living Centers
Suite 205
1501 Lee Highway
Arlington, VA 22209

(703) 243-9100

Profile: The NAILC is an independent, nonprofit organization dedicated to helping retired people and the elderly locate housing in which they can retain their independence to a large extent, despite their age, physical and mental impairments, or low income. The NAILC conducts studies in many American communities, sponsors appropriate housing legislation, and makes referrals on request to help seniors locate further information and resources at the local level.

Publications: The association publishes reports and distributes fact sheets and literature on housing for seniors.

National Association of   **NAIC**
Investors Corporation
1515 East Eleven Mile Road
Royal Oak, MI 48067

(313) 543-0612

Profile: The NAIC is a network of independent investment groups whose members invest in mutual plans of their own devising. It undertakes financial market studies through voluntary committees and provides information on investing procedures and markets in the United States. Retirees are invited to inquire about the association and its aims.

National Association of   **NARCE**
Retired Civil Employees
1533 New Hampshire Avenue
Washington, DC 20036

(202) 234-0832

Profile: NARCE is composed of former civil employees who are retired, current civil employees with five years' vested service, and their spouses. The association serves as an advocate on the part of its members, sponsoring and supporting legislation and administration regulations that are beneficial to them. NARCE invites inquiries about its programs and benefits for retired people.

Publications: NARCE publishes a newsletter and distributes free booklets and fact sheets on topics of interest to civil employees and retirees.

National Association of   **NARFE**
Retired Federal Employees
1533 New Hampshire Avenue, NW
Washington, DC 20036

(202) 234-0832

Profile: NARFE is composed of some 500,000 former federal employees who are retired, current federal civilian employees with five years' vested service, and their spouses. Since 1921, the association has sponsored and supported legislation and administration regulations that are beneficial to both present and future retirees. Information about NARFE and its benefits is available on request.

National Association of   **NASCS**
Senior Citizen's Softball
40700 Romer Plank Road
Clinton, MI 48044

Profile: The members of the NASCS are older individuals and clubs organized to promote the sport of softball. The goals of the association are to promote softball as a healthful, vigorous, and beneficial sport; to recruit men and women interested in playing it; and to set up team programs and foster competition. Inquiries are invited from experienced players and novices alike.

Publications: The association publishes a newsletter and also directories of teams, locations, and competitions.

National Association of   NASUA
State Units on Aging
Suite 304
2033 K Street, NW
Washington, DC 20006

(202) 785-0707

Profile: The role of the NASUA, as a public-interest group funded by the Department of Health and Human Services, is to provide information, technical assistance, and professional planning to state units on aging. The association also disseminates information on legislation affecting state programs on aging and services to professionals in the field of aging. Individuals can request information by contacting the NASUA branches in their states or by contacting the national office, above, for a list of state units.

Publications: Available pamphlets for the older public include *What Is a State Unit on Aging?*, *Aging America: It's Everyone's Future,* and *Model State Benefits Guide for Older Citizens.*

National Association of   NATO
Trailer Owners
Box 1418
2015 Tuttle Street
Sarasota, FL 33578

(813) 953-2730

Profile: NATO is a membership organization of the owners of trailers, campers, and motor homes, many of whom are retired, whose objective is to compare notes, arrange programs of mutual interest, and provide information to others who might want to join.

Publications: NATO publishes a magazine and a directory of overnight parks.

National Bar Association   **NBA**
1225 11th Street, NW
Washington, DC 20001

(202) 842-3900

Profile: The National Bar Association administers programs to assist the elderly with legal problems, supports community groups that provide low-cost services to those in need, and offers educational workshops on problems that especially concern older Americans. These include health issues, housing, pensions, discrimination, retirement plans, and other individual rights. The NBA also provides a referral service to help inquirers locate counseling and assistance.

Publications: The NBA publishes a professional journal and also distributes free literature on legal subjects of concern to older people.

National Bowling Association   **NBA**
377 Park Avenue
New York, NY 10016

(212) 689-8308

Profile: The National Bowling Association is the major organization in the United States dedicated to the sport of bowling. It solicits memberships, helps to form clubs and leagues, sponsors competition at all levels, establishes guidelines for instruction, and administers rules and regulations. It also supports a special program to attract older bowlers and maintains programs adapted to their levels of proficiency and ability. Inquiries are invited.

Publications: The association publishes a magazine, a newsletter, and other periodicals and distributes booklets on bowling at no cost. It also collaborates on projects for full-length books on bowling.

National Cancer Institute   **NCI**
Room 10A24, Building 31
9000 Rockville Pike
Bethesda, MD 20892

(301) 496-5583
(800) 4-CANCER

Profile: The NCI is the federal government's principal agency for underwriting cancer research and distributing information about the disease to medical and health professionals and the public. The Cancer Information Service (CIS) can provide reliable, up-to-date information about cancer and causes through the toll-free 800 number above.

Publications: The NCI distributes numerous free booklets on all forms of cancer, treatments, centers, and ways to cope with the disease, for patients and families alike.

National Caucus and   **NCCBA**
Center on Black Aged
Suite 500
1424 K Street, NW
Washington, DC 20005

(202) 637-8400

Profile: The mission of the NCCBA, as a nonprofit, voluntary agency, is to improve the quality of life for older black Americans. The caucus strengthens existing national and local organizations that provide services to older black people, conducts seminars, and advises community groups. It also encourages older blacks to volunteer for community service and helps to provide housing, jobs, transportation, and health care.

Publications: The Caucus publishes *Golden Age* magazine and a newsletter on a quarterly schedule.

National Center for   NCHPA
Health Promotion and Aging
National Council on the Aging (NCOA)
600 Maryland Avenue, SW
Washington, DC 20024

(202) 479-1200

Profile: The mission of the NCHPA is to sponsor studies and research to help the aging, serve as a clearinghouse of information for older people, support projects and legislation that benefit the elderly, sponsor senior centers and other facilities, and coordinate activities with other groups working on behalf of this constituency. The center also seeks to aid professionals who are interested in developing and implementing health promotion programs for senior citizens.

See also the National Council on the Aging, page 211.

National Center for   NCHEC
Home Equity Conversion
118 East Main Street
Madison, WI 53703

Profile: The NCHEC serves as a clearinghouse for information on home equity conversion, which sometimes can be a boon for older people who are "cash poor" but have homes that are valuable. For these people, a home equity loan (or reverse mortgage) may make it possible for them to effect an arrangement whereby they live in their homes but are paid a sum each month by an institution that is granted certain future rights to the property. The National Center for Home Equity Conversion can provide retirees and other older people with further information and referrals to institutions to which they can turn for help.

National Center for
Post-Traumatic Stress
Veterans Administration Medical Center
White River Junction, VT 05001

(802) 296-5132

See Veterans Administration, page 301.

National Center for Women
and Retirement Research
Southampton Campus
Long Island University
Southampton, NY 11968

(800) 426-7386

Profile: The mission of the center, established in 1988, is to focus exclusively on the life planning needs of women. Through research, education, and training, the center hopes to eliminate "the dismal economic situation faced by many women as they reach their later years, a situation caused by lack of income and inadequate financial knowledge and planning." Much of the emphasis is on a recent project by the Administration on Aging entitled *Pre-Retirement Education Planning for Women* (PREP), the objective being to provide expert information about ways in which women can plan better for their future and their retirement.

Publications: The center publishes guidebooks at $9.95 each, including *Looking Ahead to Your Financial Future, Social and Emotional Issues for Mid-Life Women,* and *Taking Care of Your Health and Fitness.*

National Center on Arts   NCAA
and the Aging
West Wing 100
600 Maryland Avenue, SW
Washington, DC 20024

(202) 479-1200

Profile: The NCAA is a program of the National Council on the Aging (NCOA), page 211, which seeks to stimulate more awareness of the importance of the arts as activities available to older adults and to which they can make important contributions. The center serves as a clearinghouse of information, solicits funds, and engages in studies and research aimed at providing seniors with more opportunities to participate in the arts. The NCAA also sponsors seminars and workshops, acts as a consultant to older groups interested in the arts, and maintains exhibits of the works of this senior population. Inquiries from retirees and other older men and women are encouraged.

Publications: The NCAA publishes a newsletter as well as monographs, reports, brochures, and a *Resource Guide to Persons, Places, and Programs in Arts and Aging.*

National Clearinghouse for   **NCADI**
Alcohol and Drug Abuse Information
PO Box 2345
Rockville, MD 20852

(301) 468-2600
(800) 622-HELP

Profile: The NCADI was established as an independent government agency to compile, maintain, and update the nation's largest information resource on drugs, alcohol, and substance abuse of every kind. The clearinghouse actively solicits inquiries from older men and women with drug- or alcohol-related problems, as well as from their spouses, dependents, other relatives, and close friends. The organization works closely with all other major agencies in this field.

Publications: The NCADI distributes numerous free booklets, fact sheets, and other literature on the subject and provides catalogs and references to books and audiovisual materials.

National Clearinghouse for   **NCPCI**
Primary Care Information
Suite 600
8201 Greensboro Drive
McLean, VA 22102

(703) 821-8955

Profile: This organization was established to provide information on primary care for older people. One of the objectives of such services is the delivery of ambulatory health care to urban and rural areas where there are shortages of medical personnel and facilities. The organization works largely with people in the medical and health professions and with institutions providing such care, but inquiries from seniors are invited when they need information or want referrals to local resources.

Publications: The clearinghouse publishes professional journals on the management of ambulatory care programs, but also has a list of materials of interest to individuals at no cost. One example is *Easy Eating for Well-Seasoned Adults.*

National Clearinghouse on Aging

See the National Council on the Aging, page 211.

National Committee to   NCPSS
Preserve Social Security
2000 K Street, NW
Washington, DC 20006

(202) 822-9459

Profile: The National Committee to Preserve Social Security was formed as an active lobbying and advocacy group to fight against cuts in programs and funds for Social Security, Medicare, and Medicaid. It relentlessly and aggressively campaigns at the federal level to influence members of Congress to support this battle and to vote against cuts in programs affecting older people. The committee actively solicits members and donations, and urges its members to write letters and sign petitions on behalf of these causes.

Publications: The committee publishes an official newspaper, *Saving Social Security,* and distributes fact sheets and petitionary literature to members.

National Consumers League   NCL
Suite 516
815 15th Street NW
Washington, DC 20005

(202) 639-8140

Profile: The basic roles of the NCL are to educate consumers and to bring consumer concerns and complaints to the attention of government and industry policymakers. The league works to ascertain that consumer protection programs are established and enforced. It also develops communications and programs and provides educational materials for the general public on such issues as pollution, energy, nutrition, drugs, medical and health costs, the environment, and safety.

Publications: The NCL distributes materials on the subjects mentioned above, as well as on Medicare, supplemental health insurance, nursing homes, and other services and supplies for older persons. A catalog of titles and costs is available on request.

National Council   NCAHF
against Health Fraud
PO Box 1276
Loma Linda, CA 92354

(714) 796-3067

Profile: The NCAHF was founded by a group of consumers angry at the increase in health frauds committed against the public in general and older people in particular. The council not only fights fraud but takes steps to discourage misleading promotion and advertising related to health products and programs, to set consumers straight about dietary fads, and to target doctors and other professional people who may be guilty of malpractice. The council encourages inquiries from people who know of such practices or feel they have been victimized.

National Council   **NCSC**
of Senior Citizens
1331 F Street, NW
Washington, DC 20004

(202) 347-8800
(202) 639-8513

Profile: The NCSC, an advocacy organization that is dedicated to promoting the interests of America's elderly, was founded in 1961 in the movement for Medicare, the first among many legislative achievements on behalf of seniors. Since then, the NCSC has gone on to win many more victories, including increased Social Security benefits, the creation of senior centers and nutrition sites, community employment projects, low-income senior housing, and a multitude of services under the Older Americans Act. The NCSC, which comprises over five thousand senior citizen clubs with a total membership of almost five million, encourages inquiries and membership among the retirement community.

Publications: The NCSC publishes a monthly magazine, *Senior Citizens News,* regular *Retirement Newletters,* and numerous booklets in the subject fields described above.

National Council on Alcoholism   NCA
12 West 21st Street
New York, NY 10010

(212) 206-6770

Profile: The fundamental mission of the NCA is to educate the public on all aspects of alcoholism. It works closely with health and medical professionals and with many other voluntary, non-profit organizations to enlist community support and activate its programs to combat problem drinking. Special assistance is provided to community organizations that seek to reach people who are problem drinkers and at risk of becoming alcoholics. The council also maintains an extensive library on alcoholism and related subjects. The NCA encourages inquiries from people with drinking problems, as well as from the families of alcoholics, and sponsors numerous educational and orientation programs on the subject. The NCA has branches throughout the United States, which can be contacted directly or through the national headquarters.

Publications: The NCA publishes many books and booklets on problem drinking and alcoholism and will supply a catalog of these upon request.

National Council on the Aging   NCOA
West Wing 100
600 Maryland Avenue SW
Washington, DC 20024

(202) 479-1200

Profile: The NCOA is a nonprofit membership organization for volunteers and professionals whose objective is to develop a nationwide resource for information, technical assistance, research, and training in the fields of retirement and aging. The council serves, too, as an advocate on behalf of older people in legislative matters and the development of services for seniors. It maintains an extensive library and computerized data files on aging, with the focus on medical, psychological, economic, and social aspects of growing older. The NCOA mounts an active Retirement Training Program and serves as the parent body for numerous subgroups, including the National Center on Arts and the Aging, the National Center on Rural Aging, the Senior Community Service Project, and the National Institute of Senior Centers.

Publications: The NCOA publishes and/or distributes a wide range of books and publications in its many subject fields. A list of these publications is available on request.

National Crime Prevention Council   **NCPC**
733 15th Street NW
Washington, DC 20005

(202) 393-7141

Profile: The NCPC serves as a catalyst and center of information to help American citizens prevent criminal acts and fight crime, on the streets, in the home, and elsewhere. Its services are particularly valuable to older men and women, who are often the victims of crimes, such as robberies, thefts, assaults, frauds, and con-artist schemes. The council provides professional and technical assistance to crime-fighting groups, circulates information to consumers, makes studies of criminal techniques and modes of operation, and promotes the use of methods and devices to prevent crime. The council administers the Crime Prevention Coalition, coordinates the National Citizens' Crime Prevention Campaign, and refers inquirers to local organizations for data and assistance.

Publications: The NCPC distributes free brochures, posters, and other publications to individuals and groups, and also makes available audiovisual materials and workbooks.

National Dairy Council
6300 North River Road
Rosemont, IL 60018

(312) 696-1020

Profile: Although the National Dairy Council makes available a number of free booklets and informational materials on nutrition, it is also an excellent source of data on osteoporosis. This disease, which tends to afflict older people, is caused by a lack of calcium and consequent deterioration of the bones. Upon request, the council will mail literature as well as information about audiovisual materials that are available for group instruction.

National Diabetes   **NDIC**
Information Clearinghouse
Box NDIC
Bethesda, MD 20892

(301) 468-2162

Profile: The NDIC was established by the National Institutes of Health to provide reliable data about diabetes to health professionals, patients, and the general public. The NDIC also makes available audiovisual and other instructive materials for the use of seminars and community public orientation programs. It encourages inquiries from older people who have diabetes or may be prone to this disease, and provides referrals to those seeking professional help. Special programs are directed at retirees and other elders regarding prevention, diagnosis, and treatment.

Publications: The NDIC publishes or distributes booklets on the disease, as well as a bibliography of books about diabetes.

National Digestive Diseases   **NDDIC**
Information Clearinghouse
Box NDDIC
Bethesda, MD 20892

(301) 468-6344

Profile: The NDDIC, an affiliate of the National Institutes of Health, provides information about digestive diseases to health professionals and the general public. This information makes use of printed and audiovisual materials on problems of the digestive system, such as ulcers, diarrhea, heartburn, and constipation. The NDDIC maintains a library of books, other publications, and computer files of data on this subject area.

Communications: Free booklets and fact sheets are available, including *Your Digestive System and How It Works, Digestive Health and Disease,* a directory of digestive disease organizations, and a catalog of audiovisuals.

National Education Association   **NEA**
1201 16th Street, NW
Washington, DC 20036

(202) 822-7200

Profile: The NEA, with more than two million members, is the world's largest professional association, whose ranks include teachers at all levels, faculty staff members, educational support personnel, students preparing to become educators, and retirees from all educational disciplines. The NEA was founded in 1857 "to elevate the character and advance the interests of the profession of teaching and to promote the cause of education in the United States." Many of the association's active programs and actions relate to benefits for older teachers and retirees.

Publications: In addition to periodicals and newsletters, the NEA distributes fact sheets and reports on benefits for retirees who are, or could become, members of the association.

National Executive Service Corps   **NESC**
622 Third Avenue
New York, NY 10017

(212) 867-5010

Profile: Established in 1977, the NESC is a nonprofit organization that provides management consulting assistance to other nonprofit organizations and small businesses. Its members are volunteers, largely retirees who have had experience as executives and managers with corporations, in the educational field, or as professionals. Among other things, the NESC assists retirees who have their own businesses, or are thinking of starting them, and need help.

National Eye Care Project   **NECP**
PO Box 7424
San Francisco, CA 94120

(800) 222-3937

Profile: The NECP was founded as a voluntary, nonprofit organization to provide the general public with reliable information about vision and proper care of the eyes. It disseminates information to those who request it and also serves as a referral service to help people locate eye doctors, optometrists, oculists, and other professionals in the eye care field.

National Eye Institute   NEI
9000 Rockville Pike
Bethesda, MD 20892

(301) 496-5248

Profile: The National Eye Institute, an affiliate of the National
Institutes of Health, was established to sponsor eye research, as
well as to disseminate information to professionals and consumers on the causes, prevention, diagnosis, and treatment of
eye diseases, disorders, and injuries. NEI-supported research in
medical centers in the United States investigates such matters
as the cause of blindness, the treatment of cataracts, methods
for reversing failing vision, and the early detection of glaucoma.
The NEI coordinates its activities with those of many other
health groups in presenting educational programs on the prevention of blindness.

Publications: Free booklets and fact sheets are dispensed to the
public on cataracts, glaucoma, eye care, vision impairment, and
other related topics. A list is available on request.

National Federation of   NFIB
Independent Business
Suite 700
600 Maryland Avenue, SW
Washington, DC 20024

(202) 554-9000

Profile: The NFIB is the nation's largest small-business advocacy
group, which actively lobbies on behalf of its more than 570,000
members in Washington, DC, and all fifty states. The NFIB's
areas of expertise include employee benefits, clean air legislation,

taxation and pension policies, and nonprofit government competition with the private sector. The federation also addresses itself to retirees—both in the matter of benefits and the pursuit of entrepreneurial ventures after retirement.

Publications: The NFIB issues a quarterly economic report on matters relating to independent businesses and distributes information on small business in general and the federation in particular.

National Federation of the Blind   **NFB**
1800 Johnson Street
Baltimore, MD 21230

(301) 659-9314

Profile: The NFB is the largest organization in the United States representing blind people and is committed to helping the blind and the visually impaired integrate themselves into society on an equal basis with those who are fully sighted. The NFB looks at the problems as ones that originate not from the loss of eyesight but from misunderstandings and a lack of information on the part of the public. To that end, it is dedicated to public relations programs and other communication. A specialized program is directed at the needs of the retired and senior citizens who are blind or who have severe vision problems.

Publications: The NFB distributes free literature to the public on the aforementioned issues and makes available recordings and large-print publications for those with sight loss and impairment.

National Fire Protection Association   **NFPA**
One Batterymarch Park
Quincy, MA 02269

(617) 984-7270

Profile: The NFPA is widely recognized as the international expert on fire. As publisher of *The National Fire Codes* and other standards, the NFPA is deeply involved in technical seminars and consumer education programs and is an authoritative source of consumer advice on fire prevention, protection, and safety. Of particular interest are the association's studies and programs on fire safety for retirees, shut-ins, and infirm or handicapped people. The NFPA also investigates major fires, undertakes research, and reports regularly on its findings.

Publications: The NFPA distributes numerous booklets on fire prevention and safety for older people, provides technical reports to firefighting professionals, and produces a wide variety of visual and educational materials for National Fire Prevention Week, which it sponsors each October.

National Fitness Foundation   **NFF**
Suite 412
2250 East Imperial Highway
El Segundo, CA 90245

(213) 640-0145

Profile: The goal of the NFF is to improve the general fitness of all Americans by promoting exercise programs, competition, and sports appropriate for the ages of the participants. The NFF has focused one area of its operations on programs for older people, and regularly schedules field workshops and exercises aimed at improving the fitness and health of seniors. Inquiries are invited.

Publications: The NFF publishes a newsletter and distributes free fitness booklets and program participation lists.

National Foundation for   **NFCC**
Consumer Credit
Suite 507
8701 Georgia Avenue
Silver Spring, MD 20910

(301) 589-5600

Profile: The objective of the NFCC is to establish better systems for credit and credit ratings and to provide the public with information on everything to do with establishing credit and using credit cards. The NFCC works closely with other consumer organizations in the financial field.

Publications: The NFCC produces free booklets about maintaining financial identity, selecting and using services, and knowing when to be wary about credit offers that promise a great deal but seem to require few qualifications for individual use.

National Foundation for   **NFHHC**
Hospice and Home Care
519 C Street, NE
Washington, DC 20002

(202) 547-7424

Profile: The foundation provides information to patients and their families about short- and long-term programs of health care at home and hospice care for people with terminal illnesses. Inquiries are referred to local hospice groups that can supply detailed information and assist in a care program.

See the National Hospice Organization, page 227.

National Foundation for   **NFIC**
Ileitis and Colitis
444 Park Avenue, South
New York, NY 10016-7374

(212) 685-3440
(800) 343-3637

Profile: This national foundation is dedicated to improving the quality of life for the more than two million Americans who suffer from ileitis (Crohn's disease) and ulcerative colitis. The NFIC's mission is also to increase public awareness of these disorders and to undertake research into the diagnosis, cause, and treatment for these chronic digestive problems. The NFIC maintains a special program relating to the digestive problems of older people and encourages questions and requests for information.

Publications: The NFIC prepares reports and papers on its findings, but also distributes descriptive booklets on ileitis and colitis for the orientation of laypersons.

National Foundation of   **NFDH**
Dentistry for the Handicapped
1600 Stout Street
Denver, CO 80202

(303) 573-0264

Profile: The NFDH provides information to people who need dental care but may have difficulty obtaining adequate service because they are disabled, or elderly and infirm, and unable to visit conventional dentist's offices. Inquiries are invited from persons and their families having this problem, and referrals are then made to local professionals and facilities that can help. Attention is paid to keeping costs low and avoiding traumatic mental and physical situations.

National Geriatrics Society   **NGS**
212 West Wisconsin Avenue
Milwaukee, WI 53203

(414) 272-4130

Profile: The NGS is a nonprofit educational organization whose objectives are to undertake geriatric research and to improve the quality of care given to patients who are elderly, disabled, or chronically ill. The society sponsors conferences and publishes technical literature in the field of geriatrics and acts as a clearinghouse of current data on developments in medicine, pharmacology, nursing, rehabilitation, and the social sciences. The society's public affairs office responds to inquiries about the services of institutions for elderly people and the disabled.

Publications: The NGS publishes mainly technical papers but also maintains an ongoing report on the requirements for nursing homes in all fifty states.

National Gerontology   **NGRC**
Resource Center
1909 K Street, NW
Washington, DC 20049

(202) 728-4880

Profile: This nonprofit educational organization is an arm of the American Association of Retired Persons (AARP) whose goals are to undertake geriatric research and improve the quality of care given to patients who are elderly, disabled, or chronically ill. The center serves, too, as a clearinghouse for information about aging and the aged on such subjects as retirement, health, fitness, housing, long-term care, and finances.

National Handicapped Sports   **NHSRA**
and Recreation Association
Box 33141
Farragut Station
Washington, DC 20037

Profile: The NHSRA provides information and aids in the formation of local clubs and procedures that make it possible for handicapped men and women to participate in certain sports and various forms of recreation. Individuals who are members of the association include people who are elderly and afflicted with debilitating diseases, blind and visually impaired people, deaf people, amputees, retarded people, and others with less-than-normal physical and mental capabilities.

Publications: The NHSRA publishes a newsletter and distributes publications about sports and recreation events for the handicapped, as well as calendars of events.

National Headache Foundation   **NHF**
5252 North Western Avenue
Chicago, IL 60625

(312) 878-7715
(800) 843-2256

Profile: The National Headache Foundation is a nonprofit organization that was established in 1970 and is dedicated to three basic goals: (1) to serve as an information source to headache sufferers, their families, and the physicians who treat them; (2) to promote research into potential headache causes and treatments; and (3) to educate the public to the fact that headaches are serious disorders and that sufferers need understanding and continuity of care. The NHF disseminates free information on headache causes and treatments, funds research, and sponsors public-education seminars nationwide. Special attention is given to the cause and treatment of headaches in older people, such as those caused by glaucoma and other eye disorders, arthritis, or environmental changes that take place when people retire and move to new locations.

Communications: The NHF publishes a list of practical brochures on headaches. These include *The Headache Chart, The Headache Handbook,* and *How to Talk to Your Doctor about Headaches.* Also available are audiotapes on ways to relax to relieve tensions and headaches.

National Head Injury Foundation   **NHIF**
PO Box 567
Framingham, MA 01701

(617) 879-7473

Profile: The NHIF consists of a network of two dozen regional groups whose objective is to provide information for people who have suffered head injuries and are concerned about treatment and care. One focus is on elderly people who have incurred such injuries as a result of falls. The NHIF refers callers to local facilities for detailed information and assistance. The foundation publishes an annual report and a quarterly newsletter.

National Health Information Center   **NHIC**
Department of Health and Human Services
PO Box 1133
Washington, DC 20013-1133

(202) 429-9091
(800) 336-4797

Profile: The NHIC was established to help people locate sources of specific medical and health information and professionals who can assist them. The center maintains a file of data and resources especially for older people.

See the US Department of Health and Human Services, page 292, and the National Institutes of Health, page 236.

National Hearing Aid Society   **NHAS**
20361 Middlebelt Street
Livonia, MI 48152

(313) 478-2610
(800) 521-5247

Profile: The NHAS is a nationwide professional society of hearing aid specialists whose members are dedicated to establishing codes of standards and ethics, exchanging technical information, and planning continuing education programs to help them expand their knowledge and improve their skills. The toll-free Hearing Aid Helpline, the 800 number given above, puts the public in touch with a source of information on hearing loss, hearing aids, and the location of qualified specialists in this field. The helpline, open weekdays from 9:00 A.M. to 5:00 P.M., EST, also handles consumer complaints about hearing aids.

Publications: The NHAS distributes *Facts about Hearing Aids* and fact sheets in response to questions about hearing loss and aids.

National Heart, Lung,   **NHLBI**
and Blood Institute
9000 Rockville Pike
Bethesda, MD 20892

(301) 496-4236

Profile: The NHLBI is the federal government's main agency for mounting research on diseases of the heart, lungs, and blood vessels, and the administration of blood resources. In addition to funding research programs in medical laboratories around the United States, the institute collaborates with other government agencies in the study of high blood pressure, stroke, respiratory distress, and sickle cell anemia. The NHLBI compiles and distributes information on these subjects to the general public, as well as to specialists in medical and health fields.

Publications: Publications that individuals can obtain at no cost include *A Handbook of Heart Terms, How Doctors Diagnose Heart Disease, Heart Attacks,* and *The Human Heart: A Living Pump.*

National Highway Traffic   **NHTSA**
Safety Administration
400 7th Street, SW
Washington, DC 20590

(202) 366-9550
(800) 424-9393

Profile: The NHTSA is the nation's expert on traffic safety and the federal agency responsible for motor vehicle and traffic safety issues. One of its major objectives is to impart a better understanding of the issues related to traffic and safety. To that end, it provides spokespersons, advertising, audiovisual aids, statistical charts, and a multitude of publications on such subjects as the abilities of older drivers, safety belts, automotive maintenance, impaired driving, speed enforcement, drinking and driving, motor vehicle defects, and inspections.

Publications: The NHTSA distributes the kinds of materials mentioned above at no cost to consumers and in quantity to schools and traffic safety programs.

National Hispanic Council on Aging   NHCA
2713 Ontario Road, NW
Washington, DC 20009

(202) 265-1288

Profile: The NHCA makes studies in its field and takes action to promote the well-being of older Hispanic individuals, particularly in those regions where they make up significant parts of the local population. The council provides educational materials that are linguistically and culturally appropriate for this audience and helps to train specialists and volunteers who work with older Hispanics.

Publications: Bilingual publications are produced by the NHCA on pertinent subjects such as the prevention of disease, proper nutrition, long-term care, and physical fitness.

National Home Study Council   NHSC
1601 18th Street, NW
Washington, DC 20009

(202) 234-5100

Profile: The National Home Study Council is a leading advocate of quality correspondence education in the United States. As a nonprofit organization, it serves as a clearinghouse for information about the home-study field and sponsors a nationally recognized accrediting agency that has certified more than one hundred home-study schools. For more than sixty years, the NHSC has promoted sound education and good business practices in the home-study field and has attracted many older people, especially retirees, interested in bolstering their education, working toward degrees, or simply learning about new subjects that have captured their interest. Today, more than five million Americans are enrolled in such programs, about three-fourths of them in NHSC-accredited schools.

Publications: The NHSC distributes a free directory of accredited home-study schools, as well as handbooks with a cover price, such as *Home Study Course Development Handbook,* a guide to writing courses, and *Business Standards Course,* on ethical business practices.

National Hospice Organization   **NHO**
Suite 901
1901 North Moore Street
Arlington, VA 22209

(703) 243-5900

Profile: The National Hospice Organization was formed as a means of promoting dignity and quality care for terminally ill patients and close support for their families. The NHO provides medical care and comfort for dying patients, as well as counseling for spouses and other close relatives during the most difficult periods. The organization solicits qualified volunteers and provides training for them, as well as orientation for health professionals in hospice programs. Individuals are encouraged to inquire about hospice care for themselves or relatives, both at home and in hospitals or other medical facilities.

Publications: The NHO publishes an annual directory, *Guide to the Nation's Hospices,* as well as materials to be used by volunteers and professionals who participate in hospice programs.

National Indian Council on Aging   **NICOA**
PO Box 2088
Albuquerque, NM 87103

(505) 242-9505

Profile: The NICOA, funded by the Administration on Aging, is dedicated to ensuring that older Indian and Alaskan Native Americans have ready access to comprehensive, quality health care, legal assistance, and social services in ways equal to those of other elderly groups. The council coordinates its efforts with other agencies that serve the older Native American population and conducts surveys to identify critical needs of these individuals and groups. It also serves as a clearinghouse for information about issues of concern to Native Americans and disseminates this kind of information to the public.

Publications: The NICOA publishes *Elder Voices* monthly. Free literature in this subject field is also available, including *American Indian Elderly: A National Profile.* A list is available upon request.

National Information Center on Deafness   **NICD**
Gallaudet College
800 Florida Avenue, NE
Washington, DC 20002

(202) 651-5051 (voice)
(202) 651-5052 (TDD)
(800) 672-6720 (toll-free voice and TDD)

Profile: The NICD compiles and distributes information on deafness and hearing problems to health professionals and the public. Among the materials distributed are fact sheets on aging and hearing loss, sign language, the education of people who are deaf, TDDs and other assistive devices, and data on organizations that provide services to deaf and hard-of-hearing people.

Publications: Typical of available pamphlets are *Homes and Housing for Aged Deaf Persons, Managing Hearing Loss in Later Life,* and *Aging and Hearing Loss: Some Commonly Asked Questions.*

National Injury   **NIIC**
Information Clearinghouse
USCPSC
5401 Westbard Avenue
Bethesda, MD 20207

(301) 492-6424

Profile: The NIIC was established as a center of information on all forms of injuries, to provide data for people who have suffered injuries and are concerned about treatment and care. The NIIC has made studies of the kinds of injuries most common among the elderly and serves as a clearinghouse for compiling and disseminating this kind of information. The NIIC refers inquirers to local facilities for detailed data and assistance. It also distributes publications about specific kinds of injuries, and their prevention and treatment.

National Institute of   **NIAWR**
Age, Work, and Retirement
West Wing 100
600 Maryland Avenue, SW
Washington, DC 20024

(202) 479-1200

See the National Institutes of Health, page 236, and the National Council on the Aging, page 211.

National Institute of   **NIAID**
Allergy and Infectious Diseases
9000 Rockville Pike
Bethesda, MD 20892

(301) 496-5717

Profile: The NIAID is the federal government's principal agency for research in the field of allergic and infectious diseases. The institute investigates illnesses caused by infections, as well as allergic reactions caused by insect bites, drugs, and food products. Information about this field of research is conveyed through various media to doctors, other health and medical professionals, and the general public.

Publications: Numerous free booklets and fact sheets are available on request, covering such subjects as allergies, infections, the common cold, asthma, flu, the immune system, and sexually transmitted diseases.

National Institute   **NIDR**
of Dental Research
Room 2C35, Building 31
9000 Rockville Pike
Bethesda, MD 20892

(301) 496-4261

Profile: As an arm of the National Institutes of Health, the
NIDR is the federal government's principal agency for research
on the causes, prevention, diagnosis, and treatment of conditions
and diseases of the mouth, teeth, and gums. In addition to the
central center in Bethesda, the NIDR supports a dozen dental
research centers to study tooth decay, gum diseases, and related
disorders. Special research is conducted in matters relating to
aging and to the effects of nutrition (often poor in older people)
on oral health. Information about these topics is circulated to
professional people and the public, upon request.

Publications: Free NIDR pamphlets include *Dental Tips for Dia-
betics, Fluoride to Protect the Teeth of Adults, Dry Mouth,* and
Periodontal Disease.

National Institute of Mental Health   **NIMH**
Public Inquiries
Room 11A-21
5600 Fishers Lane
Rockville, MD 20857

(301) 443-4513

Profile: The NIMH is the federal agency that supports nationwide research on mental illness and mental health. It is dedicated
to improving the mental health of the American people; fostering
the understanding, treatment, and rehabilitation of the mentally

ill; and preventing mental illness. The NIMH collects, evaluates, and disseminates statistical information on the causes, occurrence, and treatment of mental illness, trains professionals, and educates the public through the media and written publications and audiovisual materials. Among NIMH priorities are projects to identify and treat mental diseases, including Alzheimer's, in older people.

Publications: The NIMH makes numerous booklets and fact sheets available to the public at no cost. Examples of these are: *Plain Talk about Physical Fitness and Mental Health, Plain Talk about Aging, Plain Talk about Depression,* and *A Consumer's Guide to Mental Health Services.*

National Institute of Neurological   NINCS
and Communicative Disorders and Stroke
Room 8A06, Building 31
9000 Rockville Pike
Bethesda, MD 20892

(301) 496-5924

Profile: This national institute is the federal government's principal agency for research into the causes, prevention, evaluation, and treatment of neurological diseases and stroke. Studies include stroke, spinal cord injuries, tumors of the nervous system, head injuries, chronic headaches, back pain, and epilepsy—many relating to aging and elderly people. Also being researched are Alzheimer's disease, Parkinson's, Huntington's, multiple sclerosis, and ALS ("Lou Gehrig's Disease").

Publications: Reports on the above diseases and conditions are available upon request.

National Institute of Senior Centers   **NISC**
West Wing 100
600 Maryland Avenue, SW
Washington, DC 20024

(202) 479-1200

Profile: The NISC is a nonprofit organization whose members represent senior centers at the local, state, or national level—centers where older people can congregate for special services, recreation, and educational seminars on topics such as retirement, health, nutrition, housing, and financial planning. The institute upgrades existing centers and lays plans for additional ones in areas where they are needed and will be active. The NISC also establishes standards and policies and serves as an advocate for legislation to provide more benefits for seniors who attend such centers. The NISC encourages inquiries from older people, particularly retirees, on the location of centers in their areas and the types of programs they offer.

Publications: The NISC distributes descriptive literature on senior center programs and lists of locations.

National Institute of Senior Housing   **NISH**
West Wing 100
600 Maryland Avenue, SW
Washington, DC 20024

(202) 479-1200

Profile: The NISH is committed to studying the special needs of older adults for adequate housing and to implementing plans for a nationwide response to the growing demand for affordable, decent, well-designed residences for seniors, both as individuals and as groups. The institute promotes the development of community-based housing options for seniors, provides forums for the exchange of information and ideas, and represents older people as advocates in providing legislation at all governmental levels to improve housing alternatives. The NISH also serves as a clearinghouse for information about housing and residential planning for retirees and other elderly people.

Publications: The NISH publishes a newsletter, *Senior Housing News,* fact sheets and reports on senior housing plans, and a bibliography of articles and books in this subject field.

National Institute on Adult Day Care   **NIAD**
600 Maryland Avenue, SW
Washington, DC 20024

(202) 479-1200

Profile: The NIAD promotes the development of adult day care services, develops standards and guidelines, provides training for professionals and volunteers, surveys state and federal programs, and lobbies for legislation beneficial to the older people served in these centers. There are ten regional groups.

Publications: The NIAD publishes professional papers and reports and also fact sheets and booklets for laypersons on the location and role of adult day care centers.

National Institute on Aging   **NIA**
Office of Public Information
Federal Building 6C12
9000 Rockville Pike
Bethesda, MD 20892

(301) 496-1752

Profile: The National Institute on Aging is the federal government's principal agency for conducting and supporting medical, social, and behavioral research related to the aging process and the diseases and special problems of older individuals. Such research includes evaluations of Alzheimer's disease, the genetic mechanisms of aging, mental and intellectual changes that take place with age, and changes that develop in the heart, nervous system, and other organs as individuals grow older. The Office of Public Information prepares and communicates these data in a variety of ways to the general public and encourages inquiries from individuals who are concerned about any of these aspects of aging.

Publications: Free materials are available upon request on many subjects as indicated in the NIA *Publications List.* Other significant publications are the *Resource Directory for Older People, Answers about Aging, Health Resources for Older Women,* and *Age Words: A Glossary on Health and Aging.*

**National Institute on Deafness
and Other Communications Disorders
Information Clearinghouse**
9000 Rockville Pike
Bethesda, MD 20892

(301) 496-5751

See the National Institutes of Health, page 236, and the National Association for Hearing and Speech, page 195.

National Institutes of Health   **NIH**
9000 Rockville Pike
Bethesda, MD 20892

(301) 496-4000

Profile: The National Institutes of Health were established by the federal government as clearinghouses for information on major diseases and the health resources of the nation allied in the fight to prevent, diagnose, and treat these disorders. The ten institutes, located in Bethesda, Maryland, are:

National Cancer Institute

National Eye Institute

National Institute of Allergy and Infectious Diseases

National Institute of Arthritis, Diabetes, Digestive, and Kidney Disease

National Institute of Child Health and Human Development

National Institute of Dental Research

National Institute of Environmental Health Sciences

National Institute of General Medical Sciences

National Institute of Neurological and Communicative Disorders and Stroke

National Library of Medicine

National Interfaith Coalition on Aging   NICA
PO Box 1924
298 South Hull Street
Athens, GA 30603

(404) 353-1331

Profile: The coalition is composed of religious and secular groups and individuals concerned with the problems of aging and the spiritual well-being of the elderly. It promotes communications and cooperative efforts among these groups, assists churches and synagogues that respond to the needs of older people, and identifies and supports programs for the elderly that can be enhanced by religious organizations. The coalition also maintains a library on aging.

Publications: The NICA publishes a professional journal and a bimonthly newsletter for laypersons, covering the coalition's programs, calendar of events, and book reviews.

National Jewish Center for   NJCIRM
Immunology and Respiratory Medicine
1400 Jackson Street
Denver, CO 80206

(303) 398-1002

Profile: The National Jewish Center studies, researches, diagnoses, and treats respiratory, allergic, and immune system disorders. Nonprofit and nonsectarian, the center focuses on asthma, emphysema, and tuberculosis. Ground-breaking work is also being achieved with food and drug allergies, AIDS, lupus, rheumatoid arthritis, and viral infections.

Publications: The center distributes fact sheets, releases, reports, and booklets on the above-mentioned, and related, disorders.

National Kidney and Urologic   **NKUDIC**
Diseases Information Center Clearinghouse
Box NKUDIC
Bethesda, MD 20892

(301) 496-3583

Profile: The clearinghouse is an information service of the National Institutes of Health that provides information to health professionals and the public. It also maintains a computerized data bank and index covering research and programs in the field of kidney and urologic diseases.

Publications: Free publications include *Prevention and Treatment of Kidney Stones, Understanding Urinary Tract Infections, When Your Kidneys Fail: A Handbook for Patients and Their Families,* and other booklets and fact sheets of interest to laypersons.

National Kidney Foundation   **NKF**
30 East 33rd Street
New York, NY 10016

(212) 889-2210
(800) 622-9010

Profile: The NKF supports research, patient services, professional and public education, an organ donor program, and community service. Affiliates conduct community and patient services, including drug banks, transportation, early screening, and patient seminars. Individuals with questions or requests can phone the toll-free hotline, the 800 number given above, for further information.

Publications: In addition to professional journals, the foundation distributes newsletters, fact sheets, and leaflets, and makes available on loan audiovisual materials on kidney disease and treatment.

National League for Nursing   NLN
350 Hudson Street
New York, NY 10014

(212) 989-9393

Profile: The National League for Nursing is composed of some twenty thousand members in nursing and other health professions and community members who are interested in solving health care problems of many kinds. The league has special groups and committees whose focus is on the needs of retired people and the elderly, and works to assess nursing needs, home care, improved organized nursing services, education and training, and coordination between nursing and other health and community services. The NLN encourages inquiries from older people who have concerns about such matters as home care and nursing facilities.

Publications: The NLN publishes professional journals and newsletters and distributes fact sheets, memos, and leaflets on nursing. It also distributes audiovisuals and other educational materials on older people and their needs, for the use of community groups.

National Legal Aid and Defenders Association   NLADA

See Legal Services for the Elderly, page 182.

National Library of Medicine   **NLM**
8600 Rockville Pike
Bethesda, MD 20894

(301) 496-5501
(800) 638-8480

Profile: The NLM is an integral unit of the National Institutes of Health, recognized as the world's largest medical research library, containing some four million books, professional journals, visual files, and audiovisual materials in fifty biomedical subject areas. These publications and materials can be consulted at the NLM or borrowed through interlibrary loan at public libraries in most communities in the United States. The National Library also maintains computerized data bases with references to books, periodicals, and multitudes of reports and publications on every imaginable medical topic. Seven regional medical libraries coordinate activities within each region and pass requests that they cannot fulfill locally on to the NLM. Information specialists are available to answer callers on the 800-number hotline given above.

Publications: Of primary interest to laypersons is *MEDLARS: The World of Medicine at Your Fingertips,* fact sheets describing the programs and services of the library, and a list of regional medical libraries.

**National Library Service for
the Blind and Physically Handicapped**
Library of Congress
1291 Taylor Street, NW
Washington, DC 20542

(202) 707-0712

Profile: This special service for the blind and physically handicapped is administered by the Library of Congress. It makes available such media as recordings, large-print books, and other communications for people who cannot use conventional information services. Materials can be ordered and obtained through local public libraries and other organizations that focus on the problems of the blind, the visually impaired, and the handicapped. The Library of Congress encourages inquiries from the public.

National Mental Health Association   NMHA
1021 Prince Street
Alexandria, VA 22314

(703) 604-7722

Profile: The NMHA is committed to improving the mental health of the nation and to supporting studies and research on mental illness of all kinds. The association is dedicated to fighting mental disorders; fostering the understanding, treatment, and rehabilitation of the mentally ill; and preventing mental decline in the aging. The NMHA serves, too, as a clearinghouse of information on the causes, occurrence, and treatment of mental illness, and educates the public through the media and through the distribution of various publications.

Publications: The NMHA publishes a catalog, available on request, and makes numerous booklets and fact sheets available to the public at no cost.

National Motorists Association   NMA
6678 Pertzborn Road
Dane, WI 53528

(608) 849-4054

Profile: The NMA serves as an advocate for the interests of American motorists on issues ranging from transportation policies and highway maintenance to driver education, testing, traffic laws, communications, automobile insurance practices, adequate access to the justice system, and protection from warrantless search and seizure. One of the NMA's focuses is on older drivers, their needs and abilities, and legislation to protect them. The NMA is actively involved at the national and state levels, both in protecting the motorist and in lobbying for better laws. The NMA encourages contacts from older motorists.

Publications: The NMA publishes newsletters, fact sheets, and reports on its activities, many of which are of interest to retirees and other older motorists.

National Moving   **NMSA**
and Storage Association
124 South Royal Street
Alexandria, VA 22314

(703) 549-9263

Profile: The membership of the NMSA is composed of professional movers and moving companies whose objective is to improve services, determine standards for the industry, and provide better information for people who are planning to move, either with or without storing their household furniture and furnishings. The NMSA provides special information for retirees making such moves and, on request, will refer inquirers to local companies and services.

Publications: The NMSA publishes a number of free how-to booklets on such topics as planning a move, packing breakables, storage, expenses, and related activities and circumstances.

National Multiple Sclerosis Society   **NMSS**
205 East 42nd Street
New York, NY 10017

(212) 986-3240

Profile: The NMSS stimulates, supports, and coordinates research into the cause, treatment, and cure of multiple sclerosis (MS), provides services and aid for persons with MS and related disorders and their families, aids in establishing MS clinics and therapy centers, and sponsors awards to the media for reporting to the public on this subject. The NMSS maintains a library and information resource center to serve the lay public as well as professionals, and makes copies and reprints of articles and fact sheets available from these files.

Publications: The society publishes a quarterly magazine, *Inside MS,* as well as booklets about current research on the disease, coping with MS, and therapeutic advances and resources.

National Organization for   **NOVA**
Victim Assistance
1757 Park Road, NW
Washington, DC 20010

(202) 232-8560

Profile: The membership of NOVA is composed of professionals in the field of criminal justice, former crime victims, specialists who assist crime victims and witnesses, and others committed to the recognition of victims' rights. NOVA offers twenty-four-hour crisis counseling to crime victims and refers callers to supportive services throughout the United States. Special attention is given to the urgent needs of victims who are retired, elderly, or handicapped, and these people are urged to call when they need assistance. NOVA also sponsors educational programs and serves as an advocate to introduce legislation to benefit crime victims.

Publications: The *NOVA Newsletter* is published monthly. The association also publishes booklets, such as *The Elderly Crime Victim,* and other material on victims and their rights and recourses.

National Osteoporosis Foundation   **NOF**
1625 Eye Street, NW
Washington, DC 20006

(202) 223-2226

Profile: The NOF is a voluntary health agency whose members are dedicated to reducing the widespread problems of osteoporosis, a condition most often found in older women, which causes weakness in the bones and leads to increased risk of fractures. The foundation conducts studies, supports research, and inaugurates public affairs programs to increase public awareness and knowledge of the disease and methods to prevent it. Older people with concerns and questions about bone diseases can obtain information and literature from the NOF on request.

Publications: The NOF publishes a quarterly newsletter and makes consumer booklets and lists available to those who inquire. An example is *Osteoporosis: A Woman's Guide.*

National Pacific/Asian   **NPARCA**
Resource Center on Aging
410 United Airlines Building
2033 Sixth Avenue
Seattle, WA 98121

(206) 448-0313

Profile: The resource center was established as a private agency to study and improve the quality of health care and services for older people in the Pacific/Asian community. The center provides technical assistance in this field, sponsors workshops and training sessions for professionals, compiles regional data on the needs of this audience, and provides interested individuals with information about family and support groups that can assist them with their health problems and concerns.

Publications: The center produces a bimonthly newsletter, *Update*, about its programs and activities, and also maintains a *National Community Service Directory* that lists resources and publications.

National Parkinson Foundation   **NPF**
Bob Hope Road
1501 Northwest Ninth Avenue
Miami, FL 33136

(800) 327-4545

Profile: The NPF is a nonprofit organization that is affiliated with the School of Medicine of the University of Miami. Its focus is on research, diagnosis, treatment, and care of people who are afflicted with Parkinson's and other related neurological diseases. The foundation maintains continuing education and training programs for professionals and also sponsors mutual self-help groups for patients and their families, makes referrals for older people in need, and recommends treatment and rehabilitation programs for speech, physical, and occupational therapy.

Publications: In addition to professional journals and reports, the NPF distributes data sheets, reports, and leaflets to laypersons on Parkinson's, its treatment, and coping with the disease.

National Parks and   **NPCA**
Conservation Association
1015 31st Street, NW
Washington, DC 20007

(202) 944-8530

Profile: Founded in 1919, the NPCA is the only national association devoted solely to protecting and improving America's national parks. It is a private, nonprofit citizens' organization representing more than 100,000 members throughout the United States who are concerned about protection and conservation. Through speakers' programs, audiovisual materials, and publications, the NPCA discusses such park-related topics as poaching, overcrowding, acid rain, pollution, wildlife, federal land management, and special parks or park areas devoted to urban life, culture, history, and recreation. The NPCA offers special tours and discounts to senior citizens.

Publications: Numerous free publications are available for the asking, on individual national parks as well as the topics mentioned above.

National Personnel Records Center **NPRC**
ATT: Military Records
9700 Page Boulevard
St. Louis, MO 63132

(314) 263-7261 (Army)
(314) 263-7243 (Air Force)
(314) 263-7141 (Navy, Marines, Coast Guard)

Profile: The National Personnel Records Center is maintained for the use of veterans who may need their military records or data to obtain health care and other benefits. Requests for information should be made in writing except in the case of medical emergencies, when the numbers above can be called for facts and assistance. Regional offices of the Veterans Administration (VA) can also assist former military personnel. The release of information entails protective measures established by law. Relatives and next-of-kin (if the veteran is deceased) can obtain this kind of confidential information only as specified by VA regulations.

Publications: Generally, there is no charge for copies of discharge or separation papers. However, nominal fees may be charged for certain other publications and services.

National Referral Center
Library of Congress
Washington, DC 20540

(202) 287-5670
(202) 287-5683

Profile: Established in 1962, the National Referral Center is a free service of the Library of Congress that refers people with questions on almost any subject in the world—from science and engineering to the arts and humanities—to agencies that can provide the answers. In order to be able to respond to countless and continual inquiries, the center maintains and updates detailed descriptions of some fifteen thousand information resources. In addition, specialists—such as those in the field of aging, retirement, and the elderly—maintain a wealth of personal contacts to seek data on any topic not suitably covered in the conventional resource files.

Publications: Data supplied are commonly in the form of computer printouts describing the information capabilities and services of one or more organizations or resources.

National Rehabilitation Association   **NRA**
633 South Washington Street
Alexandria, VA 22314

(703) 836-0850

Profile: The membership of the NRA is composed of professionals committed to the rehabilitation of people with physical and mental disabilities. The NRA makes studies, underwrites research, and plans programs to promote therapy and independent living for people with disabilities. It also serves as an advocate to initiate legislation and facilities to benefit older people who require rehabilitative services, mounts public-education programs in this field, and encourages volunteers and training in rehabilitation counseling.

Publications: The NRA publishes *The Journal of Rehabilitation* quarterly, a *Newsletter* eight times a year, and numerous monographs, and distributes consumer literature of interest to older readers.

National Rehabilitation   **NRIC**
Information Center
8455 Colesville Road
Silver Spring, MD 20910

(301) 588-9284
(800) 346-2742

Profile: The NRIC was established as an arm of the United States Department of Education to improve the delivery of information to the rehabilitation community, as well as to the general public. The center maintains a library of books, research reports, journals, microfiche, audiovisuals, and other communications about people who are blind, deaf, developmentally impaired, emotionally disturbed, or suffering from degenerative diseases that afflict the elderly but can be treated by rehabilitative programs. The NRIC responds to inquiries from the public, supplies data, and helps refer people to local specialists and community facilities.

Publications: The NRIC publishes professional papers and also distributes newsletters, releases, and a limited number of consumer booklets on rehabilitation.

National Resource Center   **NRCCLS**
for Consumers of Legal Services
815 15th Street, NW
Washington, DC 20007

(202) 347-2203

Profile: The National Resource Center was founded as an agency to study the field and provide information for consumers seeking professional assistance and counsel on legal matters. The center acts as a clearinghouse of information for retirees and the elderly who need legal help or advice, but who have limited financial resources. The center also helps to study and evaluate various legal service plans.

Publications: The NRCCLS distributes releases, fact sheets, and reports, but also suggests sources for more detailed information on various legal subjects of concern to consumers.

National Resource Center   **NRCHPA**
on Health Promotion and Aging
1909 K Street, NW
Washington, DC 20049

(202) 728-4476

Profile: This arm of the American Association of Retired Persons (AARP) makes studies and undertakes research on the relationship between aging and health. It publishes numerous consumer booklets for AARP members and others.

See the American Association of Retired Persons (AARP), page 68.

National Retired   **NRTA**
Teachers Association
1909 K Street, NW
Washington, DC 20049

(202) 872-4700

Profile: A division of the American Association of Retired Persons (AARP), the NRTA was established to assist retired (and active) teachers to obtain more benefits and compensation, and to improve the quality of their lifestyles. Services offered include group hospital and health insurance, other forms of insurance, tax assistance, legal counsel, health benefits, consumer discounts, travel and tour assistance, and preretirement planning. Members are also eligible for discounts at certain hotel/motel chains, car rental agencies, and restaurants.

Publications: The NRTA distributes the same publications that are made available to members of AARP, as well as specialized reports, releases, newsletters, and leaflets in the field of education and teaching.

National Retiree   **NRVC**
Volunteer Center
905 Fourth Avenue, South
Minneapolis, MN 55404

Profile: The NRVC is an independent, nonprofit organization that offers retired people numerous kinds of volunteer jobs they can undertake for whatever time they have available and at their own pace. Some volunteer assignments make use of preretirement experience and specialties, while others require only the desire to serve and brief orientation periods. The NRVC welcomes inquiries.

Publications: The center publishes descriptions of volunteer jobs and lists of available positions in chosen locations.

National Retirement Concepts   **NRC**
1454 North Wieland Court
Chicago, IL 60610

(800) 888-2312

Profile: National Retirement Concepts is a private tour organization that takes groups of people ranging generally in age from forty-five to seventy to retirement cities in a number of sunbelt states—Florida, Arizona, Arkansas, and the Carolinas—on pre-views of areas in which retirees might like to live. The organization purposely avoids contact with salespeople in developments in an attempt to provide close-up samplings of communities that can then be investigated by individuals in more detail at a later date. Important parts of these preview tours are seminars with bankers, Chamber of Commerce staffers, realtors, and local government officials. Tours typically range from eight to fifteen days, with costs that are competitive with other kinds of vacation tours in the same regions. Older people who are retired or are planning retirement can obtain information from the NRC (and two or three other similar tour operators) but should be specific about their interests and desire to avoid salespersons and high-pressure promotions.

National RV Owners Club	**NRVOC**

PO Drawer 17148
Pensacola, FL 32522

(904) 477-2123

Profile: The membership of the NRVOC is composed of vehicle owners, dealers, manufacturers, campground administrators, and others with a stake in recreational vehicles. The objectives of the club are to provide service and technical information, initiate and support legislation advantageous to owners and users, review and evaluate RV products, and provide training programs and RV-use workshops. The club is also active in organizing tours and rallies, sponsoring contests, and providing assistance for RV participants with problems. Considerable focus is placed on the needs of retirees and older people because of the high proportion of RV owners who are in this category.

Publications: The club publishes a magazine, *Living the RVing Lifestyle,* newsletters, member profiles, and fact sheets on RV use and travel.

National School Volunteer Program   **NSVP**
Suite 320
701 North Fairfax Street
Alexandria, VA 22314

(703) 836-4880

Profile: The NSVP promotes the involvement of individuals and groups in educational programs in their communities. It assists schools in establishing workable volunteer programs and is considerably interested in soliciting the help of retirees and older people who have had experience in the educational field or are dedicated to the improvement of school facilities and programs. State and local affiliates of the NSVP provide training for volunteers in such subject areas as basic skills, English as a second language, and special education. Would-be volunteers are urged to contact the program.

Publications: The NSVP publishes a newsletter covering its activities and the opportunities for volunteer participation.

National Second Opinion   **NSOP**
Program (Surgery)
Room 1503
52 Vanderbilt Avenue
New York, NY 10017

(212) 370-7820
(800) 522-0036

Profile: The NSOP serves individuals seeking second-opinion consultations from surgeons on the necessity of proposed surgery. Its objective is to contain medical costs and avoid unnecessary expense. The program seeks to heighten patients' awareness as consumers of medical services and focuses much attention on the needs and medical services of older people. Concerned patients and their families can obtain help through the NSOP hotline, the 800 number given above.

Publications: The NSOP has published a book on the subject, *Second Opinion Elective Surgery,* and issues reports on surgery and alternate treatments.

National Self-Help Clearinghouse   **NSHC**
City University of New York
Room 620
25 West 43rd Street
New York, NY 10036

(212) 642-2944

Profile: The NSHC does not have a membership but is a clearinghouse of information on self-help groups. It provides a referral service, conducts research, promotes training activities, and maintains a speakers' bureau.

Publications: The NSHC publishes a quarterly, *Self-Help Reporter,* a newsletter, and brochures.

National Senior Citizens Law Center   **NSCLC**
Suite 700
1052 West Sixth Street
Los Angeles, CA 90017

(213) 482-3550

Profile: The NSCLC is a legal services support center specializing in the legal problems of the elderly. It acts as an advocate on behalf of elderly people with low incomes in litigation and administrative affairs. The center also sponsors conferences and workshops on aspects of the law affecting the elderly. It responds to inquiries from the public.

Publications: The center publishes a weekly newsletter, a monthly magazine on nursing homes, handbooks, and guides.

National Senior Sports Association   NSSA
10560 Main Street
Fairfax, VA 22030

(703) 385-7540

Profile: The membership of the NSSA is composed of men and women fifty and older who are active in sports and recreational activities. It helps older Americans maintain their health and fitness through sports, and conducts regional and national senior tournaments in bowling, golf, and tennis. It also offers travel programs and a Member Exchange File whereby traveling members can contact other members to enjoy sports together.

Publications: The NSSA publishes *Senior Sports News* monthly.

National Shared Housing   NSHRC
Resource Center
6344 Greene Street
Philadelphia, PA 19144

(215) 848-1220

Profile: The role of the NSHRC is to provide information, education, specialized assistance, and research on shared housing. To that end, it provides counsel, technical help, speakers, and regional training workshops on planning and developing group-residence programs. The center works as an advocate toward the removal of financial, legal, and restrictive measures against shared housing, and bestows awards in recognition of housing programs that have been judged creative and positive.

Publications: The center publishes *Shared Housing Quarterly*, a newsletter for consumers, and numerous professional reports, releases, and recommendations.

National Society to   **NSPB**
Prevent Blindness
79 Madison Avenue
New York, NY 10016

(800) 221-3004

Profile: The NSPB is committed to preserving sight and preventing blindness by sponsoring community education programs, developing local services, and supporting research. It distributes information about eye care and safety, vision deficiencies and diseases, and the location of medical facilities specializing in the diagnosis and treatment of vision problems. Local chapters offer specific tests for individuals, including those for glaucoma and the disabilities of older people. The society sponsors LIFESIGHT: Growing Older with Good Vision, an educational program for older people.

Publications: The NSPB publishes and disseminates numerous booklets on eye safety, glaucoma, vision tests, and other pertinent subjects.

National Stroke Association   **NSA**
Suite 240
300 East Hamden Avenue
Englewood, CO 80110-2622

(303) 762-9922

Profile: The NSA provides information about the nature of stroke, its diagnosis, and treatment to the general public and makes technical data available to professionals. The association also offers assistance and support to patients and their families, serves as a clearinghouse for information, sponsors research, and encourages self-help services for people recovering from strokes. It responds to inquiries from patients and their families in this respect and provides guidance for people forming stroke clubs and other support groups.

Publications: The association distributes *Open Channels* quarterly and publishes numerous brochures for laypersons. Examples are *Stroke: What It Is, What Causes It, Proper Diet after Stroke,* and *The Road Ahead: A Stroke Recovery Guide.*

National Urban League   **NUL**
500 East 62nd Street
New York, NY 10021

(212) 310-9000

Profile: The NUL, composed of some fifty thousand members, is a voluntary, nonpartisan community service agency of professional, business, civic, and religious leaders with a staff of trained social workers. Its mission is to eliminate racial segregation and discrimination, and to achieve parity for minority groups in all walks of life. Its activities extend into such fields as housing, education, transportation, health, family life, labor, law, veterans' affairs, social welfare, and retirement planning. The Seniors in Community Service Program provides training and part-time employment for low-income persons fifty-five and older. The NUL encourages retirees to get in touch and volunteer.

Publications: Free publications include *Quick Facts about the Urban League Movement,* as well as reports, fact sheets, and releases on the league's fields of activity.

National Victim Center   **NVC**
Suite 1001
307 West Seventh Street
Fort Worth, TX 76102

(817) 877-3355

Profile: The NVC leads the nationwide fight for the rights of crime victims, serving as a national resource center for more than seven thousand victim advocacy and criminal justice organizations. The center addresses issues regarding abuse of the elderly, as well as child abuse, sexual assault, domestic violence, crime, and racial attacks. Older people with concerns and problems as victims should contact the center for referral to local specialists and facilities that can help them.

Publications: The NVC distributes fact sheets, reports, and releases on the many topics relating to victims and their rights and resources.

National Wheelchair   **NWAA**
Athletic Association
1604 East Pikes Peak Avenue
Colorado Springs, CO 80909

(303) 632-0698

Profile: The NWAA is composed of members who are athletes but have been disabled by polio, spinal cord injuries, amputation, or problems caused by aging. Their primary mission is to ready themselves to compete in various amateur sports events in wheelchairs. Among the sports in which NWAA members compete are softball, track and field events, archery, swimming, table tennis, slalom, and weight lifting. Older people with disabilities are especially encouraged to inquire about sports and competition in these fields.

Publications: The NWAA publishes a newsletter, sports programs and entry forms, and rule books.

North Carolina Center
for Creative Retirement
University of North Carolina
Asheville, NC 28800

Profile: The North Carolina Center for Creative Retirement is a new program developed by the University of North Carolina to encourage older participants who are interested in developing activities that are more stimulating and rewarding. As yet, there has been no formal establishment of programs and procedures, and there are no ongoing publications. Retirees and people planning retirement are encouraged to inquire about current activities and future plans. The northwestern region of North Carolina has become increasingly popular as a location for retirement, with a favorable mix of climate, scenery, facilities, activities, and people.

ODPHP National Health Information Center
PO Box 1133
Washington, DC 20013-1133

(301) 565-4020
(800) 336-4797

See the National Health Information Center, page 224.

Office for Civil Rights   OCR
Department of Health and Human Services
330 Independence Avenue, SW
Washington, DC 20201

(202) 245-0188

Profile: It is the responsibility of the Office for Civil Rights to enforce federal laws prohibiting discrimination against persons because of their age, sex, race, color, national origin, faith, handicap, or other condition. Older people who feel they have been discriminated against for one or more of these factors should contact the Office for Civil Rights as soon as possible. Regional offices are located in Boston, New York City, Philadelphia, Atlanta, Chicago, Dallas, Kansas City, Denver, San Francisco, and Seattle, as well as Washington, DC.

Office of Consumer Affairs   **OCA**
Room 5718
Department of Commerce
Washington, DC 20230

(202) 377-5001

Profile: The Office of Consumer Affairs is charged with overseeing all areas of activity that relate to the consumer. In this respect,
it serves as a source to which older people can turn when they
have complaints about consumer products and services.

Office of Fair Housing and Equal Opportunity   **OFHEO**
Room 5100
451 Seventh Street
Department of Housing and Urban Development
Washington, DC 20410

(202) 755-7252
(800) 424-8590

Profile: The Office of Fair Housing and Equal Opportunity serves
as a watchdog for all areas of housing, and particularly seeks to
avoid discrimination of any kind against people because of age,
sex, color, race, national origin, or faith. Older people who feel
that they were discriminated against in the matter of housing can
turn to this agency for assistance.

Office of Human Development Services   **OHDS**
200 Independence Avenue, SW
Washington, DC 20201

(202) 245-0724

See the Administration on Aging, page 50.

Office of Minority   **OMHRC**
Health Resource Center
PO Box 37337
Washington, DC 20017-37337

(301) 587-1938

Profile: The OMHRC was established to compile information, undertake studies, and disseminate information about diseases and disorders that particularly affect minority groups, including blacks, American Indians, Eskimos, and Hispanics. Older people in these categories can seek special assistance through the center if they are afflicted with such illnesses.

Publications: The center publishes a list of brief leaflets and fact sheets relating to specific diseases and treatments.

Office of Special Education   **OSERS**
and Rehabilitative Services
Room 3132, Switzer Building
330 C Street, SW
Washington, DC 20202-2524

(202) 732-1241

Profile: The OSERS assists in the education of people of all ages who have problems with disabilities. Although originally founded as an agency to assist the young, it has spread into the areas of the retired as more and more older people become involved with educational programs and in many cases are restricted by disabilities and handicaps. The OSERS is also directly involved with agencies that provide programs for the blind, the deaf, and others who have visual or auditory impairments.

Publications: The OSERS publishes numerous brochures, reports, and newsletters in conjunction with agencies and educational institutions that have special teaching programs for the handicapped.

Office on Smoking and Health   OSH
Room 1-16, Park Building
5600 Fisher's Lane
Rockville, MD 20857

(301) 443-1690

Profile: The OSH, as an agency of the Public Health Service, compiles and circulates information on the health risks that are associated with smoking. It also recommends methods for giving up smoking, conducts regular surveys on smoking habits, and supports educational programs on the relationship between smoking and the development of various diseases. A program for older people and retirees is of current interest.

Publications: The OSH publishes many technical bulletins on research and the health consequences of smoking and also a number of consumer brochures on the health risks, how to stop smoking, and antismoking legislation.

Older Women's League   OWL
Suite 300
730 11th Street, NW
Washington, DC 20001

(202) 783-6686

Profile: The Older Women's League was formed to eradicate the inequities faced by women—particularly those in midlife and older—in many walks of life. The national agenda established by OWL consists of seven advocacy and education issues: Social Security reform, pension rights, job discrimination, access to health care, family caregivers, federal budget priorities, and staying in control of one's life until its end. Local OWL chapters provide mutual aid and supportive services to older women, especially those who are alone, provide testimony before legislatures, communicate with the media on women's rights, host seminars and workshops to orient professionals and lay volunteers, and work to improve the economic situation of older women. OWL solicits volunteers and encourages older women in need to contact local branches for information and assistance.

Publications: The league publishes the *OWL Observer* monthly, as well as a number of other publications such as *Aging and Health, Health Care in Retirement,* and *Gray Papers.*

Oral Health Research Center   **OHRC**
110 Fuller Place
Hackensack, NJ 07601

(201) 692-2622

Profile: The Oral Health Research Center is an independent, nonprofit organization whose mission is to study all aspects of oral health, provide training to professionals, and communicate with the public.

Publications: The center distributes fact sheets and literature on the care of the teeth and the mouth.

Paralyzed Veterans of America   **PVA**
801 18th Street, NW
Washington, DC 20006

(202) 872-1300
(800) 424-8200

Profile: This association of some fifteen thousand members is composed of military veterans who have incurred an injury or disease that caused paralysis. The mission of the PVA is to obtain Veterans Administration benefits due the members, to work toward federal benefits of various kinds, to provide aid in securing jobs, housing, and training, and to plan retirement for members who are sixty and older. Nonmembers who might qualify are urged to make inquiries of the PVA and to enroll in the program.

Publications: The PVA publishes *Paraplegia News,* a magazine reporting on the organization's efforts to ensure better care for paralyzed veterans and their families. It also distributes material in booklet form on pertinent subjects relating to paralysis and disability.

Parkinson's Education Program   **PEP**
1800 Park Street
Newport Beach, CA 92660

(714) 640-0218
(800) 344-7872

Profile: PEP compiles, catalogs, and distributes information on Parkinson's disease and related disorders, produces and lends audiotapes about symptoms and treatments, and circulates data to the press and the public to increase the general understanding of this perplexing condition.

Publications: PEP distributes fact sheets and releases on diet, exercise, and the organization of support groups to aid patients and their families.

Pension and   **PWBA**
Welfare Benefits Administration
Office of Program Services
Department of Labor
Third Street and Constitution Avenue
Washington, DC 20216

(202) 523-8921

Profile: The PWBA is the source to which older people can turn for information and assistance when they are planning retirement and are concerned about any aspect of pensions and welfare benefits.

Publications: The administration publishes professional papers and reports but also distributes leaflets to consumers on pensions, welfare rights, and related topics, upon request.

Pension Rights Center   **PRC**
Suite 305
1701 K Street, NW
Washington, DC 20006

(202) 296-3778

Profile: The PRC is a public-interest group whose goal is to protect and promote the pension rights of retirees, workers, and their families, and to find practical solutions to the nation's retirement income problems. The PRC acts as an advocate to represent the interest of retirees and workers before various government agencies and to support legislation that benefits older workers and retirees.

Publications: The center publishes a newsletter as well as booklets and fact sheets on pension issues.

Pharmaceutical Manufacturers   **PMA**
Association
1100 15th Street, NW
Washington, DC 20005

(202) 835-3400

Profile: The PMA is a private organization of manufacturers of brand-name pharmaceutical, prescription, and biological products established to engender better public recognition of the industry and its products. The association also lobbies on behalf of the industry and circulates information on policies and regulations that affect its members. Although the PMA is an industry-related body, consumers can contact it and expect a response if they have valid and serious complaints about pharmaceutical products and cannot obtain satisfaction through other channels.

Publications: The PMA produces consumer booklets on prescription drugs and related products and maintains a membership list to which consumers can refer.

Philanthropic Advisory Service   **PAS**
Council of Better Business Bureaus
1515 Wilson Boulevard
Arlington, VA 22209

(703) 276-0100

Profile: The Philanthropic Advisory Service is a department of the Council of Better Business Bureaus (CBBB), dedicated to alerting consumers to fraudulent practices and scams in the field of philanthropies. The CBBB solicits complaints from consumers about such frauds, and provides information about specific agencies and institutions upon request. Since older people are often the target of questionable philanthropies, this contact is often useful.

Publications: The CBBB publishes numerous consumer leaflets and fact sheets on these, and related, topics.

Presidential Greetings Program
Greetings Office
The White House
Washington, DC 20500

Profile: An unexpected surprise to give on a wedding anniversary or birthday to someone who has reached a ripe old age is a presidential greeting. The program, which originally was intended only for elders who had reached 100, is now available for anyone who is eighty or older or celebrating a wedding anniversary of fifty years or more. If you are interested in obtaining a presidential greeting for someone who fits either category, write at least thirty days in advance to the Greetings Office. This service is administered by volunteers, most of whom are senior citizens themselves.

President's Council on   PCPFS
Physical Fitness and Sports
Suite 7103
450 Fifth Street, NW
Washington, DC 20001

(202) 504-2064

Profile: The PCPFS was established as a catalyst for communicating to the public the importance of good health and fitness and encouraging exercise and sports programs for Americans in all walks of life. The council makes recommendations and works closely with other organizations in this field, such as the Association for Fitness in Business (AFB). The council encourages participation by older men and women and acts as a referral service to put them in touch with organizations that can be helpful.

Publications: The PCPFS newsletter is published six times a year. Council publications for older people include *The Fitness Challenge in the Later Years* and *Walking for Exercise and Pleasure.*

Public Health Service   **PHS**
5600 Fishers Lane
Rockville, MD 20857

(301) 443-2404

See the United States Department of Health and Human Services, page 292.

Public Policy Institute   **PPI**
1909 K Street, NW
Washington, DC 20049

(202) 638-6815

Profile: The Public Policy Institute is a branch of the American Association of Retired Persons (AARP), established to study the position of older people in America and resolve policies and procedures that will be beneficial to seniors and recognize their rights. Through the PPI, retirees can obtain referrals to organizations that can be of assistance in many fields of activity.

Publications: AARP publishes more literature, from fact sheets and pamphlets to full-length books, than any other organization devoted to the interests of the elderly and the retired. A catalog of publications is available on request.

Project Share   **PS**
129 Jackson Avenue
Hempstead, NY 11550

(516) 485-4600

Profile: The mission of Project Share is to match compatible senior citizens in house-sharing arrangements in Nassau County, New York, working in coordination with the Family Service Association. Through interviews, Project Share social workers find and introduce potential homeowners and tenants. Even though Project Share is limited in the area it serves, the agency has provided advice and referrals to individuals and groups nationwide.

Public Service Commission   **PSC**
450 Fifth Avenue, NW
Washington, DC 20001

(202) 626-5110

Profile: The PSC serves as a body to oversee the operations and policies of individual public utility companies across the nation. It provides information, referrals, and contacts for people who may have problems with any aspect of public utilities, or who may require special assistance. Many utilities, for example, have programs for older people to help them with the payment of bills. Most, too, have energy conservation programs that older people should know about.

Publications: Booklets are available on energy conservation and the maintenance of heating and air-conditioning equipment and other utilities in the home.

Railroad Retirement Board   **RRB**
Room 556, Suite 500
2000 L Street, NW
Washington, DC 20036

(202) 653-9536

Profile: The RRB provides service to employees and retirees covered under the Railroad Retirement Act, and to their spouses or
survivors. They can assist inquirers by answering questions about
annuities, explaining benefits, providing insurance claim forms,
and helping solve any retirement problems that exist. Most states
have one or more Railroad Retirement Board district offices,
which can be located in the telephone directory.

Publications: The RRB publishes a directory of district offices
and also makes available numerous informational booklets on
such topics as retirement, pensions, insurance, and benefits.

Recorded Periodicals
919 Walnut Street
Philadelphia, PA 19107

(215) 627-4230

Profile: This service makes available all kinds of recordings for the
blind and the visually impaired.

Recordings for the Blind
20 Roszel Road
Princeton, NJ 08540

(609) 452-0606
(800) 221-4792

Profile: Recordings for the Blind is a nonprofit, voluntary organization that provides books on tape on a loan basis for people who are blind or visually impaired.

Rehabilitation International   **RI**
25 East 21st Street
New York, NY 10010

(212) 420-1500

Profile: This nonprofit organization is composed of national and international groups that conduct rehabilitation programs for people with physical and mental handicaps in some eighty countries. It serves as a world clearinghouse for information dealing with all phases of disabilities, their prevention, treatment, and rehabilitation. A special program is focused on the needs of older people who require rehabilitation.

Publications: The organization publishes a directory of worldwide services in this field and distributes booklets in many languages on rehabilitation programs.

Rehabilitation Services Administration   **RSA**
Department of Human Services
Room 1111
605 G Street, NW
Washington, DC 20001

(202) 727-3227

Profile: The RSA is the unit of the federal government responsible for overseeing the nation's rehabilitation services and programs. Its main value to retirees, the elderly, and other individuals requiring rehabilitation is to serve as a clearinghouse of information and to provide referral service to local agencies that can assist.

Publications: The RSA publishes a directory of rehabilitation services and centers throughout the United States.

Retired Enlisted Association   **REA**
14305 East Alameda Avenue
Aurora, CO 80040

(303) 364-8737

Profile: The membership of the REA is composed of men and women who are retired from the military service and who were in the enlisted ranks during their tours of duty. The association is opened to retirees who served with the army, navy, air force, marines, coast guard, and certain other government organizations that work closely with the armed forces.

Publications: The REA publishes a monthly journal and circulates newsletters and bulletins on subjects of interest to armed forces retirees.

Retired Officers Association   **ROA**
201 North Washington Street
Alexandria, VA 22314-2529

(703) 549-2311

Profile: Membership in the ROA includes men and women who are, or have been, commissioned as officers or warrant officers in any component of the armed forces—army, navy, marines, air force, and coast guard, or the National Oceanic and Atmospheric Administration. The ROA supports a strong national defense and represents and assists members and their families with benefits and retirement issues. It sponsors social services, travel, insurance, educational, and retirement employment programs, and conducts seminars.

Publications: The ROA publishes a monthly magazine, *The Retired Officer,* as well as newsletters and reports on military-related topics.

Retired Persons Services   **RPS**
One Prince Street
Alexandria, VA 22314

(703) 684-0244

Profile: This organization is a service established by the American Association of Retired Persons (AARP) to provide both prescription and nonprescription drugs by mail order at discount prices. RPS centers also offer vitamins, health-care accessories, and other medical/health products. The centers are in twelve states, where they also provide walk-in service.

Publications: The RPS regularly publishes a catalog of products available, with updated price lists, and a directory of its local pharmacies.

Retired Professional Action Group

See the Gray Panthers, page 165, which absorbed this group into its own program.

Retired Senior Volunteer Program   RSVP
806 Connecticut Avenue, NW
Washington, DC 20525

(202) 634-9353

Profile: The RSVP program—volunteers sharing the skills of a lifetime to support their communities by helping others—is an important resource for many American communities that are hard pressed to meet the needs of their residents. RSVP members are volunteers sixty and older from all socioeconomic levels who are willing and able to perform services on a regular basis. RSVP brings people of retirement age more fully into community life through their involvement with other people. Projects involve many diverse settings, such as schools, churches, the courts, health care centers, day care agencies, youth centers, retirement centers, hospitals, and many other institutions.

Publications: RSVP distributes leaflets and fact sheets on its programs and related activities.

International Action: An international program (RSVPI) can be reached at 200 Madison Avenue, New York, NY 10016, (212) 686-7788.

Retirement Research Foundation   **RRF**
Suite 214
1300 West Higgins Road
Park Ridge, IL 60068

(312) 823-4133

Profile: The RRF is a private body composed of members who are dedicated to developing programs to improve the quality of life for retired people and the elderly. The RRF sponsors service programs in various communities to enable older people—whether singles or couples—to live more independently. It works to upgrade the quality and extent of long-term care and nursing home facilities, and it awards grants to support organizations that provide employment opportunities and active volunteer programs for retired people.

Publications: The RRF does not distribute consumer booklets but does publish an annual report and statements of policy.

Road Runners Club of America   **RRCA**
629 South Washington Street
Alexandria, VA 22314

(703) 836-0558

Profile: The RRCA is a private association of people who are interested in striving for physical fitness through running and other vigorous exercises. The club is composed of people of all ages and solicits inquiries and membership from older people who are fit and want to remain that way. Awards and prizes are offered for competitive meets.

Publications: The RRCA publishes a newsletter and distributes literature on the benefits of running, walking, and similar activities.

Ross Laboratories
Department 106730-S1
Nutrition Services
Columbus, Ohio 43216

(614) 227-3065

Profile: Ross Laboratories is a manufacturer of nutritional products and protein supplements for the health field and professional use and can answer inquiries about nutritional services for older people.

Publications: Ross Laboratories publishes a directory, *Long-Term Care and Geriatric/Gerontological Associations,* and a number of useful leaflets, including *Long-Term Care Currents, Geriatric Medicine Currents,* and *Dietetic Currents.*

Rural Information Center   **RIC**
Room 304
National Agricultural Library
Beltsville, MD 20705

(301) 344-2547

Profile: The RIC is a branch of the National Agricultural Library that serves as an information center for people who live in rural communities. One section of the library is devoted to the health, welfare, and living conditions of retirees and the elderly who live in rural sections of the United States. The library responds to requests for information from retired people.

Publications: The center distributes information about its holdings and materials that are available to the general public.

Salvation Army   **SA**
National Headquarters
799 Bloomfield Avenue
Verona, NJ 07044

Local phone numbers can be found in most telephone directories.

Profile: The Salvation Army, founded in 1865, is an international religious and charitable movement that was organized and operated on a quasi-military pattern. The motivation of the SA is love of God and a practical concern for the needs of humanity. Its mission is to disseminate Christian truths, supply basic human necessities, provide personal counseling, and undertake the regeneration and rehabilitation of people in need, regardless of age, sex, creed, race, or color. The Salvation Army is continuously concerned about the welfare of older people and has developed many programs to assist them. It brings meals to individuals' homes, visits shut-ins, sponsors community education programs, offers counseling on family matters and financial problems, and will, in fact, tackle just about any problem that older people face. The SA actively solicits older volunteers to work in its programs in all parts of the United States, as well as in just about every other country in the world.

Publications: The Salvation Army produces and distributes publications on a multitude of subjects. Examples of several of particular interest to retirees are: *Do You Need a Will?*, *Confidential Record of Personal Financial Affairs*, *Friends of the Army*, *How Do You Own Your Property?*, *Gifts to Minors*, and *Trusts and Power of Attorney*.

Select Commission on Aging   **SCA**
United States House of Representatives
G-41 Dirksen Building
Washington, DC 20510

(202) 224-5364

Profile: The Select Commission on Aging was established as a body to review the needs of older people in relation to legislation and governmental facilities and programs and recommend changes and improvements for the welfare of those concerned. Information about the SCA can be obtained by writing to your senator or representative in Washington, either for general data or facts and findings about specific issues.

Publications: Reports and findings by the commission are matters of public record and available through members of Congress or members of the commission itself.

Self-Help Center   **SHC**
Suite S-122
1600 Dodge Avenue
Evanston, IL 60201

(312) 328-0470

Profile: The Self-Help Center serves as a clearinghouse for the compilation and dissemination of information on all types of self-help groups. The center organizes mutual consultancy workshops to bring laypersons and professionals together with self-help group representatives. The center conducts seminars and sponsors research on the effectiveness of self-help groups, some of which relate to retired people and the elderly.

Publications: The center publishes an annual *National Directory of Self-Help Groups,* as well as brochures, workbooks, and articles on self-help and mutual aid.

Self-Help for   **SHHHP**
Hard-of-Hearing People
4848 Battery Lane
Bethesda, MD 20814

(301) 657-2248

Profile: The members of the SHHHP are hard-of-hearing people and their families, professionals working with hearing-impaired persons, and volunteers. The organization educates members and the public about the causes and treatment of hearing loss, its detection, management, and possible prevention or cure. It develops public awareness of the problems associated with hearing loss and researches alternate methods of communication. The association responds to inquiries from individuals and solicits volunteers from the ranks of the retired, particularly those who are themselves hearing impaired.

Publications: In addition to professional journals, the SHHHP distributes leaflets and reprints of articles on self-help for hearing losses.

Senior Community Service   **SCSEP**
Employment Program
Department of Labor
Third Street and Constitution Avenue
Washington, DC 20216

(202) 535-0522

Profile: The SCSEP, administered at the federal level by the
Department of Labor and now affiliated with the American Association of Retired Persons (AARP), is designed to provide part-
time jobs in community service for unemployed, low-income
individuals who are fifty-five or more, with priority given to those
in their sixties and older. The SCSEP administers projects in all
fifty states and US territories. These are sponsored by state governments and the following national organizations: AARP, Green
Thumb, National Council of Senior Citizens, National Council on
the Aging, National Urban League, National Caucus and Center
on Black Aged, and National Association for the Hispanic Elderly.

Publications: Leaflets, reports, fact sheets, and other publications
are available through the SCSEP or the organizations listed above.

Senior Companion Program   **SCP**
1100 Vermont Avenue, NW
Washington, DC 20525

(202) 634-9351

Profile: Administered by ACTION, the Senior Companion Program is based on the simple idea that the best way to help people
is to help them help each other. In this spirit, the SCP draws on
volunteers who are themselves sixty or over, with low incomes,
who wish to establish a meaningful relationship with other older
persons, particularly the frail elderly in their homes. The SCP

also provides services to elderly people in institutions in an attempt to enable them to return to community life.

Publications: The SCP publishes a directory and distributes fact sheets and reports on its activities.

Senior Enhancing Lifelong Fitness Program   SELF
Idaho State University
Pocatello, ID 83209

(208) 236-3620

Profile: The SELF program is a unit of the University of Idaho's research program on retirement and aging. It makes studies in this field, funds research, sponsors community educational seminars, and provides information to older individuals who are interested in improving their lifestyle as they grow older and remaining as healthy and active as possible. The university responds to requests for further information on SELF.

Publications: The public relations office of the university circulates releases, articles, and reports on the program and its accomplishments and findings.

Service Corps of Retired Executives   SCORE
Suite 503
1825 Connecticut Avenue, NW
Washington, DC 20009

(202) 653-6279

Profile: SCORE, which was launched by the Small Business Administration (SBA) in 1964, provides the American entrepreneur with an important commodity: counseling and training based on years of actual business experience. SCORE is composed of fourteen thousand men and women from all walks of business management, most of them retired, who volunteer their time and talent in some 750 counseling locations throughout the United States, Puerto Rico, and Guam. SCORE counselors receive no pay for their services, though they are reimbursed for authorized travel expenses through the SBA, and the recipients pay no fees. SCORE supplies information to retirees starting their own businesses and helps set up counseling sessions. It also recruits retirees who are qualified and interested in volunteer work.

Publications: SCORE publishes descriptive brochures about its services and related activities.

Seventy-Plus Ski Club
104 East Side Drive
Ballston Lake, NY 12019

(518) 399-5458

Profile: The club was founded by a group of senior skiers and accepts members who are seventy years or older only. For a membership fee of $5.00, they receive a card, a patch, and an eleven-page list of ski areas that offer either free skiing or substantial discounts to the group. The club encourages skiers seventy or over to join the seven thousand seniors from North America, South America, Europe, and New Zealand who are now members.

Publications: In addition to the directory, the club publishes and mails two newsletters, one in June and one in November.

Skin Cancer Foundation   **SCF**
245 Fifth Avenue
Suite 2402
New York, NY 10016

(212) 725-5176

Profile: The Skin Cancer Foundation is a nonprofit educational organization whose mission is to keep the public informed about various forms of skin cancer, its prevention and treatment. It provides specialized information about skin cancers in older people, and it encourages people of all ages to avoid harmful exposure to the sun. The foundation helps teach people how to recognize and act on early warning signs of skin cancer; it sponsors screening clinics for that purpose and makes referrals to specialists in this field.

Publications: SCF publishes a newsletter and free brochures about the dangers of sun exposure, symptoms, and treatment. Posters are also available. A list of SCF materials is available on request.

Small Business Administration   **SBA**
Office of Consumer Affairs
1441 L Street, NW
Washington, DC 20416

(202) 653-6170

Profile: The Small Business Administration was established as a government body to study small-business practices and opportunities, conduct research, inform the public, and sponsor educational programs and workshops for people who owned small businesses or were considering starting them. The SBA serves as an advocate in promoting legislation that benefits such ventures. Detailed programs are devoted to entrepreneurs who are retired, to women, and to other special-interest groups. The SBA works closely with volunteers such as the Service Corps of Retired Executives (SCORE), which advises owners and managers of small businesses. It encourages retirees to volunteer their services as well.

Publications: The SBA produces numerous self-help guides, directories, and educational publications for owners or potential owners of small businesses.

Social Security Administration   SSA
Office of Information
Room 4-J-10, West High Rise
6401 Security Boulevard
Baltimore, MD 21235

(301) 965-1234
(800) 234-5772

Profile: The Social Security Administration is the agency of the federal government responsible for all the aspects of Social Security, including retirement income, health care, and survivors and disability programs. The SSA pays benefits to retired, ill, or disabled workers and their eligible spouses and other dependents, as well as to eligible survivors of deceased workers. Supplemental Security Income payments are available to individuals who have disabilities, are blind, or are needy and sixty-five or older. Older persons will find Social Security offices listed in every telephone directory in the United States, usually under the Federal or United States headings.

Publications: The SSA publishes and distributes numerous free booklets and directories on its services, including *Social Security . . . How It Works for You,* and *What You Should Know about Medicare.*

Society for Advancement   **SATH**
of Travel for the Handicapped
Suite 1110
26 Court Street
Brooklyn, NY 11242

Profile: The SATH was founded as a private, nonprofit service to make studies and provide information and assistance for people who are handicapped and want to enjoy travel, whether at home or abroad. The society sponsors seminars on travel for people with physical disabilities of all kinds, and enlists the cooperation of airlines, steamship lines, railroads, bus companies, other carriers, and terminals in providing helpful facilities. It also serves as an advocate to institute federal and state legislation to benefit handicapped people while they are traveling. Inquiries are encouraged from retired people, the elderly, and others who need such assistance.

Publications: The SATH distributes literature counseling readers on better ways to travel and cope with handicaps.

Society for Nutrition Education   **SNE**
Suite 900
1736 Franklin Street
Oakland, CA 94612

(415) 444-7133

Profile: This organization is composed of nutrition educators from the fields of dietetics, public health, home economics, industry, and education whose mission is to promote nutritional well-being for the public. The SNE has programs for older people and sponsors seminars and other public-education programs directed at this audience. The society responds to inquiries from consumers.

Publications: The SNE publishes a professional journal and distributes consumer leaflets on nutrition topics.

Society for the Right to Die   SRD
250 West 57th Street
New York, NY 10107

(212) 246-6973

Profile: The SRD promotes the rights of people to plan dignified deaths when faced with terminal illness and incurable, debilitating diseases. The society provides information and referrals for patients and their families, sponsors public-education programs, and works closely with other organizations in this and related fields, such as hospice.

Publications: The society publishes a newsletter and distributes booklets and fact sheets to the public.

State Insurance Regulators
Superintendent of Insurance
614 H Street, NW
Washington, DC 20001

(202) 727-7424

Profile: Each state in the union has a commissioner or other appointed official who is responsible for overseeing the laws and regulations governing all forms of insurance within the state. A primary function of the state regulatory agencies is to protect your interests as an insurance policyholder, particularly when you have complaints or problems that cannot be resolved through the individual insurance companies concerned. Foremost among these services are counseling programs for retired and elderly people. State agencies are listed in telephone directories under State Government headings.

Publications: These agencies publish regular newsletters or fact sheets, as well as information about scheduled workshops and seminars.

Talent Bank

See the Volunteer Talent Bank, page 305.

Tax-Aide Program   TAP
AARP Program Department
1909 K Street, NW
Washington, DC 20049

(202) 728-4455

Profile: The Tax-Aide Program (TAP) was established as a source of information and assistance for older people. Among other things, it helps with the preparation of federal income tax returns for people who are incapacitated or otherwise unable to tackle the job effectively.

Travel Assistance International   TAI
1133 15th Street, NW
Washington, DC 20005

(800) 821-2828

Profile: The TAI was established as a service for retirees and older people to provide information and assistance, and to make referrals about travel, whether domestic or foreign. The program is particularly focused on tours, facilities, and procedures to assist older travelers who have physical or mental handicaps that make travel difficult.

Union College   **UCALL**
Academy for Lifelong Learning
Wells House
Schenectady, NY 12308

(518) 370-6172

Profile: The UCALL program was established in 1988 as a membership organization for older people who wish to continue learning in an intellectually stimulating environment. Members share with others their expertise and interests, whether as planners, instructors, committee participants, or enthusiastic learners. Membership is open to all individuals who want to learn with their peers, regardless of the extent of their formal education or degrees. Besides on-campus courses, benefits also include films, theater, exhibits, concerts, lectures, and access to Union College recreational, sports, and cultural facilities.

Publications: UCALL publishes information about programs, as well as a newsletter describing numerous campus and off-campus events.

United Seniors Health Cooperative   **USHC**
Suite 500
1334 G Street, NW
Washington, DC 20005

(202) 393-6222

Profile: United Seniors is a cooperative of older persons working together to achieve better health, increased independence, and more financial security. The USHC regularly develops and offers innovative programs and services to inform consumers on health care issues. It also uses the power of its membership to improve the quality and reduce the costs of health care for older Americans. Members receive discounts on home care services, eye examinations and glasses, dental care, hearing tests, podiatry, and chiropractic services. The cooperative conducts professional seminars to help its members on such subjects as medical record keeping, Medicare benefits, long-term care, and legal issues such as living wills and durable power of attorney.

Publications: The USHC publishes a bimonthly newsletter as well as brochures and reports on long-term care, health benefits, shared housing, nursing care, insurance, and other pertinent topics.

United States Badminton Association   **USBA**
501 West Sixth Street
Papillion, NE 68046

(402) 592-7302

Profile: The USBA is the governing body for the sport of badminton and establishes regulations and assists in the development of clubs and associations. It has established information programs for older people interested in the sport and assists them in finding local clubs and events suited to their age and skills.

United States Fire Administration   **USFA**
16825 South Seton Avenue
Emmitsburg, MD 21727

(301) 447-1080

Profile: The mission of the USFA is to make studies of fires that occur in the United States (more than eighty thousand every day!) and provide the public with information about taking precautions to prevent most of these fires. The USFA conducts seminars and workshops for professionals and the public alike, responds to requests for information, and maintains a special program for older people who are incapacitated or would have difficulty escaping fires in their places of residence.

Publications: The USFA publishes numerous booklets on fire safety, such as *Let's Retire Fire.*

United States Golf Association	USGA

United States Golf Association   **USGA**
PO Box 708
Far Hills, NJ 07931

(201) 234-2300

Profile: The USGA serves as the governing body for golf in the United States, provides extensive data on the sport, and assists in planning and administering tournaments and promoting professional golf schools. The USGA maintains many special programs for players over sixty-five, and responds to requests for information from this segment of the golf-playing population.

Publications: The USGA publishes *Golf Journal* and numerous other booklets on the sport, as well as handbooks, regulation and rule books, and teaching manuals.

United States Government

Departments and agencies that can provide retirees and other older Americans with information, assistance, publications, educational programs, and referrals:

United States Chamber of Commerce
1615 H Street, NW
Washington, DC 20062
(202) 659-6000
Business and commercial enterprises

United States Department of Agriculture
Human Nutrition Information Service
6505 Belcrest Road
Hyattsville, MD 20782
(301) 436-7725
Foods, nutrition, and health supplements

United States Department of Health and Human Services
Room 4760
330 Independence Avenue, SW
Washington, DC 20201
(202) 245-0188
Health, education, retirement, programs for older people

United States Department of Housing and Urban Development
2104 HUD Building
451 Seventh Street, NW
Washington, DC 20410
(202) 755-6422
Housing, residential alternatives for older people

United States Department of Labor
Room N 4659
Third Street and Constitution Avenue, NW
Washington, DC 20216
(202) 523-8921
Pension and welfare benefits, employment for older people

United States Department of State
Citizens Emergency Center
2201 C Street, NW
Washington, DC 20520
(202) 647-5225
Assistance during emergencies when out of the country

United States Department of Transportation
400 Seventh Avenue, SW
Washington, DC 20590
(202) 366-4000
Transportation facilities for older people and the handicapped

United States Equal Employment Opportunity Commission
2401 E Street, NW
Washington, DC 20507
(202) 634-6922; (800) 872-3362
Complaints about discrimination of any kind

United States Food and Drug Administration
HFE-50
5600 Fishers Lane
Rockville, MD 20857
(301) 443-1719
Complaints about foods and food costs

United States Forest Service
Human Resources Programs
1375 K Street, NW
Washington, DC 20013
(202) 535-0927
*Special programs and discounts for older people visiting national
parks, monuments, and campgrounds*

United States Health Resources and Services Administration
5600 Fishers Lane
Rockville, MD 20857
(301) 443-2086
*Information and assistance relating to any aspects of health and
older people*

United States Office of Consumer Affairs
614 H Street, NW
Washington, DC 20201
(202) 727-7000
Complaints about consumer products and services

United States Postal Services
ATT: Chief Postal Inspector
Washington, DC 20260-2100
(202) 245-5445
Complaints about junk mail or mail fraud

United States Securities and Exchange Commission
Public Reference Branch
Stop 1-2
Washington, DC 20549
(202) 272-7440
Information about securities and investments, and complaints about suspected securities frauds and scams

United States League of   **USLSI**
Savings Institutions
111 East Wacker Drive
Chicago, IL 60601

(312) 644-3100

Profile: The USLSI provides information on savings institutions and facilities of all kinds and distributes literature on savings plans and related topics.

United States National Senior Sports Organization   USNSSO

Suite N-300
14323 South Outer Forty Road
Chesterfield, MO 63017

(314) 878-4900

Profile: The USNSSO is a nonprofit organization whose goal is to promote fitness and physical excellence through competition among people fifty-five and older. Working toward this objective, the USNSSO assists local communities in strengthening already existing senior games and establishing new senior games, and works closely with the media, national sponsors, and other sports organizations to increase the awareness and support of senior games.

Publications: The USNSSO publishes a directory of senior games, as well as fact sheets and numerous releases about its programs.

United States Tennis Association   USTA

1212 Avenue of the Americas
New York, NY 10036

(212) 302-3322

Profile: The USTA is a federation of tennis clubs, educational groups, recreational departments, individuals, and others interested in the promotion of tennis and its development as a means of healthful recreation and physical fitness. The association sanctions thousands of tennis tournaments for all ages and develops special programs and matches for older players.

Publications: The USTA publishes a special yearbook, several tennis magazines and newsletters, and many other books and pamphlets.

United States Tour Operators Association   USTOA
Suite 12-B
211 East 51st Street
New York, NY 10022

(212) 944-5727

Profile: The membership of the USTOA is composed of individuals and organizations in the tour industry. In recent years, the association has studied, implemented, and promoted special tours for people who are older or incapacitated in any way. It responds to requests for information from people in this category.

United Way of America   UW
Headquarters
95 M Street, NW
Washington, DC 20024

(202) 488-2000

Profile: The United Way is an association of local, independent agencies in some 2,500 cities and towns in the United States and Canada. Most of the local agencies, which are funded through contributions from individuals and groups and largely staffed by volunteers, include ongoing programs for older people, the nature and degree depending upon the conditions, situations, and financial status of those in need. The UW responds readily to requests from older people about either volunteering in programs or being assisted with benefits.

Communications: The UW distributes a number of booklets and fact sheets on its programs and several videotapes, including *The Graying of America* and *The United Way and You.*

University of Iowa
Health Center Information and Communication
283 Medical Laboratories Building
University of Iowa
Iowa City, IA 52242

(319) 335-8037

Profile: The health center is a clearinghouse for information about consumer health, retirement, aging, and other subjects of particular interest to older people. Much of this data derives from the university's Geriatrics Education Center, which studies and releases information on such topics as long-term care, the problems of aging, Alzheimer's disease, nutrition, chronic conditions common in older people, osteoporosis, selecting a family physician in a new community, vision impairment, organ transplants, major diseases, new breakthroughs in medical research, and many other subjects. Inquiries are encouraged from seniors.

Publications: The health center regularly distributes releases and fact sheets on the topics mentioned above and many more.

University Research Associates   **URA**
Research Park
Arizona State University
7855 South River Parkway
Tempe, AZ 85284

(602) 839-4493

Profile: The URA is a research center whose greatest interest to older people is its distribution of information about breakthroughs in medicine and improved health care for older people. The center can be contacted for factual information, reports on health and medicine, and referrals to other sources of data and assistance.

Vacation and Senior Citizens Association   **VSCA**
15th Floor
275 Seventh Avenue
New York, NY 10001

(212) 645-6590

Profile: The VSCA serves as a coordinator and information clearinghouse for several hundred senior citizens centers and vacation camps. It makes studies and reports on changes in existing programs and the development of new programs, provides educational assistance to professional staff members in this field, and offers a referral service for older people interested in knowing more about facilities, locations, and programs. The VSCA absorbed two other programs of this nature, Vacations for the Aging and the Association of Senior Centers.

Publications: The VSCA maintains an updated list of centers and camps and publishes a brochure.

Vacation Exchange Club   **VEC**
Youngtown, AZ 85363

(602) 972-2186

Profile: The membership of the VEC is composed of individuals, couples, and families who are interested in exchanging their places of residence temporarily with other people similarly inclined. The exchange club serves as a link between these people and coordinates its activities with other home-exchange groups in the United States and an increasing number of countries abroad.

Publications: The club publishes a semiannual *Exchange Book,* a directory of some six thousand families seeking exchange and travel arrangements.

Vegetarian Society   **VS**
PO Box 926
Joshua Tree, CA 92252

(619) 366-2478

Profile: The Vegetarian Society disseminates information to the general public about vegetarian diets. Inquiries from older people who are on vegetarian diets or interested in them are invited.

Veribank, Inc.
PO Box 461
Wakefield, MA 01880

(800) 442-2657

Profile: Veribank is an independent bank research firm that specializes in assessing the safety and strength of the country's federally insured financial institutions, savings and loan associations, commercial banks, credit unions, and insurance companies. Using financial data filed with bank regulators, Veribank applies automated analysis techniques to determine which institutions meet its standards of asset quality, capital strength, earnings, liquidity, and other objective criteria. Veribank provides written reports by mail or instant ratings by phone. Information and fees are available on request.

Publications: Veribank publishes a newsletter, *The Banking Safety Digest,* data sheets, news releases, booklets like *Know Your Bank,* and a book, *Is Your Money Safe?* ($3.95).

Vestibular Disorders Association   **VDA**
Suite D-230
1015 Northwest 22nd Avenue
Portland, OR 97210-3079

(503) 229-7705

Profile: The VDA was founded in 1983 as an organization dedicated to achieving the following goals: providing a support network for people with dizziness and balance disorders, maintaining
a resource center for information and services, educating the
public and health professionals about vestibular disorders and
their effects, and supporting research programs to improve the
quality of life for people afflicted with these disorders. The VDA
makes studies of problems that particularly affect older people,
and it encourages inquiries from this segment of the population.
It supports educational seminars and workshops and provides a
referral service for individuals and their families interested in
knowing where to turn in their community for further information and assistance.

Communications: The VDA produces books, booklets, newsletters, directories, and videotapes, which may be purchased or
borrowed.

Veterans Administration   **VA**
810 Vermont Avenue, NW
Washington, DC 20420

(202) 233-4000

Also:
Veterans Affairs Medical Center
St. Louis, MO 63125

(314) 894-6534

Profile: The Veterans Administration was established in 1930 to administer laws authorizing benefits for former members of the armed forces and their dependents. Examples of these benefits include compensation for disabilities or death related to military service; pensions based on financial need for totally disabled veterans, whose handicaps were not related to service in certain instances; education and rehabilitation; home loan mortgages; burial; and a medical program involving clinics, medical centers, and nursing homes. Toll-free numbers for the VA are listed in local telephone directories under U.S. Government.

Publications: Federal Benefits for Veterans and Dependents is published and updated regularly by the VA to describe the benefits mentioned above and other related programs and facilities.

Veterans of Foreign Wars   **VFW**
200 Maryland Avenue, NE
Washington, DC 20002

(202) 543-2239

Profile: The VFW is a two-million-member service organization that was established more than ninety years ago, after the Spanish-American War, to represent the common interests of men and women who served, whether at home or abroad, in foreign wars. The VFW maintains a nationwide network of some ten thousand local posts and, through its service officers, directly assists veterans and their dependents in obtaining benefits. Many of the association's activities are, of course, beneficial to retirees and other older Americans. Listings for the VFW can be found in most telephone directories.

Publications: The VFW publishes a magazine and distributes releases, fact sheets, and newsletters, many of them through local posts.

Villers Foundation
Suite 3
1334 G Street, NW
Washington, DC 20005

(202) 628-3030

Profile: The mission of the Villers Foundation, formed in 1982, is to foster fundamental changes in institutions and attitudes affecting the elderly. Priority areas include health care, income security, and the contributory roles played by older people in society. Special focus is directed toward seniors who are members of minority groups or have low incomes. The primary thrust of the foundation is to provide grants to assist local and statewide groups to advocate and organize activities that encourage lower-income seniors to take better charge of their lives. The foundation invites recommendations from older people about locations and activities that could benefit from such grants.

Publications: The foundation publishes an annual report and professional papers on its activities and grants.

Vision Foundation   **VF**
812 Mount Auburn Street
Watertown, MA 02172

(617) 926-4232
(800) 852-3029

Profile: The Vision Foundation was formed in 1970 by several women who were visually impaired but not legally blind. Because they had progressive eye diseases, they wanted to prepare themselves for blindness by sharing information and providing emotional support to one another. Their initial enterprise has expanded into the work of this private, self-help organization whose services now include support groups, an information clearinghouse, a referral center, a "buddy" telephone network, and the Visually Impaired Elders Network. This VIEN program offers free in-home service for seniors whose vision is failing but who are not legally blind, and provides rehabilitation services on a short-term basis. One of its major objectives is to encourage these people to be independent. Inquiries are encouraged through the toll-free 800 number given above, which answers with a taped message after hours and on weekends.

Publications: The Vision Foundation publishes a resource book, *Coping with Sight Loss,* which is updated annually, a resource list, and bimonthly newsletters.

Vitamin Information Bureau   **VIB**
664 North Michigan Avenue
Chicago, IL 60611

(312) 751-2223

Profile: The Vitamin Information Bureau is a private, for-profit organization that distributes information on the role of vitamins and minerals in maintaining health and fitness. It responds to inquiries and provides specialized data for older people who have nutritional problems or deficiencies.

Volunteer Lawyers Project   **VLP**
American Bar Association
1800 M Street, NW
Washington, DC 20049

(202) 331-2297

Profile: The VLP program is staffed by lawyers and others in the legal profession who volunteer their professional time and services free to help the elderly, the poor, and the disadvantaged. Older people who are in need of assistance are encouraged to contact the American Bar Association for further information, assistance, and referrals.

Volunteers of America   **VOA**
3813 North Causeway Boulevard
Mezaire, LA 70002

(504) 837-2652

Profile: Founded in 1896, Volunteers of America is a nonprofit ministry of service that helps people in need in more than two hundred communities across the United States. The agency's special concerns include homelessness, drug addiction, alcoholism, care of the elderly, rehabilitation of prisoners, adoption and child care, and care of the mentally and physically handicapped. Programs that focus on older people's needs include Meals-on-Wheels, transportation, homemaker assistance, and household repairs and maintenance. The VOA also sponsors foster grandparent programs and helps older people obtain day care, group residences, and nursing home care. Retirees are encouraged to apply as volunteers.

Publications: The VOA publishes booklets describing its services and opportunities that are available to volunteers.

Volunteer Talent Bank   **VTB**
1909 K Street, NW
Washington, DC 20049

(202) 872-4700

Profile: The VTB is a computerized referral project that matches volunteers who are fifty or older with available positions and fields of opportunity. The American Association of Retired Persons (AARP), which administers the program and will accept volunteers who are not AARP members, recognizes that retirees can make significant contributions to the development, support, and expansion of an organization's program. With this in mind, it has opened up new roles and opportunities for volunteers and encourages inquiries from older Americans who would like to serve.

Publications: The Volunteer Talent Bank provides listings of areas in which volunteers are needed, supplies registration forms, and distributes leaflets, article reprints, and fact sheets on opportunities for volunteer service.

Volunteer: The National Center   **VNC**
Suite 500
1111 North 19th Street
Arlington, VA 22209

(703) 276-0542

Profile: Founded in 1979, Volunteer seeks to encourage more people to undertake voluntary assignments to strengthen existing programs or assist in launching new ones. The VNC assists communities in reinforcing, expanding, and improving the effectiveness of their voluntary activities. It maintains a network of some four hundred affiliated volunteer centers and provides training for professionals and nonprofessionals alike. The VNC communicates with the public through numerous media, sponsors National Volunteer Week, and presents awards for special service. Retirees and other older people are especially welcome as prospective volunteers.

Publications: The center produces an annual catalog of available publications, a magazine on volunteering, and a newsletter describing people and activities in this field.

Walker's Club of America   WCA
437 Golden Isles Drive #15E
Hallandale, FL 33009

(305) 456-6182

Profile: The WCA, which has been in operation since 1911, is an umbrella group with affiliated clubs nationwide. Its mission is to educate the public about the benefits of walking for exercise and fitness and as a stimulating form of competition. The club plans and conducts walking seminars and events nationwide and provides a complete program of events for sponsors.

Publications: The WCA maintains a list of walking clubs and related organizations, which it will mail upon receipt of a stamped, self-addressed #10 envelope (4" × 9½").

Walking Association   WA
PO Box 37228
Tucson, AZ 85740

(602) 742-9589

Profile: The Walking Association is composed of individuals who are interested in walking for exercise and physical fitness and who would like to increase and improve routes and facilities for walking. The group's members exchange suggestions and ideas and act as advocates for legislation to establish more, and safer, walkways. The association encourages retirees to consider membership and become involved in walking programs and events in their communities.

Publications: The association publishes guides and manuals and a quarterly newsletter.

Women's Equity Action League   **WEAL**
Suite 305
1250 Eye Street, NW
Washington, DC 20005

(202) 898-1588

Profile: The membership of WEAL consists of individuals and groups whose objective is to secure better economic, legal, and social rights for women. The league serves as an advocate to lobby for and support legislation in this respect. It conducts research, publishes reports, promotes educational workshops and seminars for professionals and laypersons, and distributes information about career counseling and training programs for women. WEAL maintains active programs for women who are retired and encourages participation by older women.

Publications: Among the many publications distributed by WEAL are *Equal Opportunity for Women, Women and Sports,* and *Women and Education.* It also publishes fact sheets on insurance, taxes, Social Security, and discrimination.

World Peace Foundation   **WPF**
22 Batterymarch Street
Boston, MA 02109

(617) 482-3875

Profile: The World Peace Foundation is a private organization whose goal is to advance the cause of peace through public education. The WPF conducts studies of characteristic international problems and communicates its findings through the media, publications, and seminars. Areas of study, for example, have been United States–Latin America relationships and international economic conflicts. From a demographic viewpoint, the WPF has also focused on problems of older people, and welcomes inquiries from retirees interested in participating in world peace movements.

Publications: The World Peace Foundation reports on its studies and circulates releases and article reprints on topics related to this field of investigation.

World Wildlife Fund   **WWF**
1250 24th Street, NW
Washington, DC 20037

(202) 293-4800

Profile: The World Wildlife Fund is an organization devoted to the solicitation of contributions to assist in the preservation of wildlife, particularly endangered species, throughout the world. The fund encourages older people, especially those who are retired and seeking programs that need volunteers, to offer their time and expertise to assist in the cause of wildlife protection.

Young Men's Christian Association   **YMCA**
101 North Wacker Drive
Chicago, IL 60606

(312) 977-0031

Profile: Although the YMCA has traditionally been associated with young people, it has changed considerably over the years and now offers a number of programs for senior citizens, such as day care for the elderly and classes for older people with various kinds of disabilities. Retirees and other older people with time on their hands are invited to investigate the "Y" as an opportunity for voluntary work as well as a source of personal assistance in time of need.

Publications: The YMCA produces many books and other publications, including directories, magazines, newsletters, and fact sheets. A copy of its annual directory is available upon request.

Young Women's Christian Association   **YWCA**
726 Broadway
New York, NY 10003

(212) 614-2700

Profile: Like the YMCA, the YWCA has changed considerably over the years in the types of people it attracts and enlists for volunteer work. Not only are more women involved but they tend to be older and more concerned with serious issues impacting on retirement, housing, health, legal matters, and financial patterns. Would-be volunteers are urged to contact local offices of the YWCA for information.

Publications: The YWCA publishes informational brochures on a wide range of subjects, for which a catalog is available upon request.

BIBLIOGRAPHY

The following books and publications will be helpful to anyone wishing to know more about the subject areas highlighted here:

General

AARP Worker Equity Department. *Think of Your Future: Preretirement Planning Workbook.* Des Plaines, Ill.: Scott, Foresman and Company, 1986.

Attwood, William. *Making It through Middle Age.* New York: Atheneum, 1982.

Averyt, Anne C. *Successful Aging.* New York: Ballantine Books, 1987.

Butler, Robert N. *Why Survive? Being Old in America.* New York: Harper & Row, 1985.

Chapman, Elwood N. *Comfort Zones: A Practical Guide for Retirement Planning.* Los Altos, Calif.: Crisp Publications, 1985.

Comfort, Alex. *A Good Age.* New York: Crown, 1978.

Fischer, David H. *Growing Old in America.* New York: Oxford University Press, 1977.

Fries, J. F., and L. M. Crapo. *Vitality and Aging.* San Francisco: W. H. Freeman, 1981.

Georgakas, D. *The Methuselah Factors: Strategies for a Long and Vigorous Life.* New York: Simon & Schuster, 1980.

Haber, Carole. *Beyond Sixty-five: The Dilemma of Old Age in America's Past.* New York: Cambridge University Press, 1983.

Hallowell, C. *Growing Old, Staying Young.* New York: William Morrow & Co., 1985.

Henig, Robin M. *Myth of Senility.* Des Plaines, Ill.: Scott, Foresman and Company, 1988.

Monroe, Mary Ellen. *The Challenge of Aging: Bibliography.* Littleton, Colo.: Libraries Unlimited, 1983.

Palder, Edward L. *The Retirement Source Book.* Kensington, Md.: Woodbine House, 1989.

Skinner, B. F., and M. E. Vaughan. *Enjoy Old Age.* New York: Norton, 1983.

Tournier, Paul. *Learn to Grow Old.* New York: Harper & Row, 1983.

Selecting Retirement Areas

AARP. *Your Home, Your Choice: A Workbook for Older People and Their Families.* Washington, DC: AARP, 1990.

Bowman, Thomas F., George Giuliani, and Ronald Minge. *Finding Your Best Place to Live in America.* Dixville, NY: Red Lion Books, 1982.

Boyer, Richard, and David Savageau. *Places Rated Retirement Guide.* Chicago: Rand McNally, 1983.

———. *Places Rated Almanac.* Chicago: Rand McNally, 1985.

Dickinson, Peter. *Travel and Retirement Edens Abroad.* Des Plaines, Ill.: Scott, Foresman and Company, 1983.

———. *Sunbelt Retirement: Complete State by State Guide.* Des Plaines, Ill.: Scott, Foresman and Company, 1986.

———. *Retirement Edens Outside the Sunbelt.* Des Plaines, Ill.: Scott, Foresman and Company, 1987.

Dunlop, Richard. *On the Road in an RV.* Des Plaines, Ill.: Scott, Foresman and Company, 1988.

Franke, David, and Holly Franke. *Safe Places for the Eighties.* New York: Dial Press, 1984.

Gold, Margaret. *Guide to Housing Alternatives for Older Citizens.* Mount Vernon, NY: Consumer Reports Books, 1985.

Houston Chamber of Commerce. *Inter-City Cost-of-Living Index.* Houston: American Chamber of Commerce, 1990.

Manser, Nancy. *Older People Have Choices: Information about Health, Home and Money.* Minneapolis: Augsburg, 1984.

Shattuck, Alfred. *The Greener Pastures Relocation Guide.* Englewood Cliffs, NJ: Prentice-Hall, 1984.

Sumichrast, Michael, Marika Sumichrast, and Ronald Shafer. *Planning Your Retirement Housing.* Des Plaines, Ill.: Scott, Foresman and Company, 1984.

Medicine and Health

AARP. *Prescription Drug Handbook.* Des Plaines, Ill.: Scott, Foresman and Company, 1990.

Alpert, Joseph, M.D. *The Heart Attack Handbook.* Boston: Little, Brown & Co., 1984.

American Medical Association. *Family Medical Guide.* New York: Random House, 1982.

Arthritis Foundation. *Understanding Arthritis.* Mount Vernon, NY: Consumer Reports Books, 1984.

Benowicz, Robert. *Vitamins and You.* New York: Berkley Books, 1984.

Berland, Ted. *Fitness for Life.* Des Plaines, Ill.: Scott, Foresman and Company, 1987.

Brecher, Edward M. *Love, Sex, and Aging.* Mount Vernon, NY: Consumer Reports Books, 1984.

Brody, Jane. *Jane Brody's Nutrition Book.* New York: Bantam, 1982.

———. *The New York Times Guide to Personal Health.* New York: Times Books, 1982.

Butler, R., and Myrna Lewis. *Love and Sex after 60.* New York: Harper & Row, 1977.

———. *Aging and Mental Health.* St. Louis: C. V. Mosby, 1989.

Callender, Sheila. *Blood Disorders.* New York: Oxford University Press, 1986.

Chaitow, Leon. *New Help for Arthritis.* Rochester, Vt.: Thorsons, 1987.

Consumer Group. *Prescription Drugs.* Belfast, Me.: Porter, 1985.

Consumer Information Center. *Headaches.* Pueblo, Colo.: Consumer Information Center, 1984.

Coombs, Jan. *Living with the Disabled: You Can Help.* New York: Sterling, 1984.

Dartmouth Medical School. *Medical and Health Guide for People over 50.* Hanover, NH: Dartmouth Institute, 1990.

Fitzgerald, Kathleen. *Alcoholism: the Genetic Inheritance.* New York: Doubleday, 1988.

Foner, A., and K. Schwab. *Aging and Retirement.* Monterey, Calif.: Brooks/Cole, 1981.

Hale, Gloria, ed. *Sourcebook for the Disabled.* New York: Holt, Rinehart and Winston, 1982.

Hartmann, Ernest, M.D. *The Sleep Book.* Des Plaines, Ill.: Scott, Foresman and Company, 1986.

Hausman, Patricia. *Foods That Fight Cancer.* New York: Warner Books, 1985.

Henig, Robin. *How a Woman Ages.* New York: Ballantine Books, 1985.

Hickey, T. *Health and Aging.* Monterey, Calif.: Brooks/Cole, 1980.

Horne, Jo. *Caregiving: Helping an Aging Loved One.* Des Plaines, Ill.: Scott, Foresman and Company, 1985.

Kirkpatrick, Jean. *Turnabout: New Help for the Alcoholic Woman.* Seattle: Madrona, 1986.

Koff, Theodore H. *Hospice: A Caring Community.* Boston: Little, Brown & Company, 1980.

Krop, Thomas, and Gerald Aldhizer. *The Doctor's Book on Hair Loss.* Englewood Cliffs, NJ: Prentice-Hall, 1983.

Lavin, John H. *Stroke: From Crisis to Victory: A Family Guide.* Danbury, Conn.: Franklin Watts, 1985.

Lazlo, John. *Understanding Cancer.* New York: Harper & Row, 1987.

Long, James W., M.D. *Essential Guide to Prescription Drugs: What You Need to Know for Safe Drug Use.* New York: Harper & Row, 1985.

Lonneth, Richard, and Gale Kumchy. *Back to Normal: Living Your Life to Prevent Back Pain.* New York: Doubleday, 1986.

Lucas, Jerry, and Harry Lorayne. *Memory Book.* New York: Ballantine Books, 1985.

Mace, Nancy L., and Peter V. Rabins. *The 36-Hour Day.* Baltimore: Johns Hopkins University Press, 1982.

Macheath, Jean. *Activity, Health, and Fitness in Old Age.* New York: St. Martin's Press, 1984.

Mamatos, Imanuel. *The No Hair-Loss Hair Care Book.* Englewood Cliffs, NJ: Prentice-Hall, 1988.

Manser, Nancy. *Older People Have Choices: Information about Health, Home, and Money.* Minneapolis: Augsburg, 1984.

Margolies, Cynthia. *Understanding Leukemia.* New York: Scribner's, 1987.

Markson, E. *Older Women.* Lexington, Mass.: D. C. Heath, 1983.

Meyer, Louis. *Off the Sauce.* New York: Macmillan, 1986.

Nassif, Janet Zhun. *The Home Health Care Solution.* Mount Vernon, NY: Consumer Reports Books, 1985.

Palmer, Paige. *The Senior Citizen's 10 Minutes a Day Fitness Plan.* Babylon, NY: Pilot Books, 1984.

Powell, Lenore, and Katie Courtice. *Alzheimer's: A Guide for Families.* Reading, Mass.: Addison-Wesley, 1983.

Prudden, Bonnie. *After Fifty Fitness Guide.* New York: Villard Books, 1986.

Roth, Jay S. *All about Cancer.* Philadelphia: George F. Stickley, 1985.

Shea, Timothy, and Joan Smith. *Over Easy Foot Care Book.* Des Plaines, Ill.: Scott, Foresman and Company, 1987.

Skinner, B. F., and M. E. Vaughan. *Enjoy Old Age.* New York: Norton, 1983.

Sorvino, Paul. *How to Become a Former Asthmatic.* New York: New American Library, 1986.

Starr, Bernard, and Marcella Weiner. *The Starr-Weiner Report on Sex and Sexuality in Mature Years.* New York: McGraw-Hill, 1982.

Vaughan, Clark. *Addictive Drinking: The Road to Recovery.* New York: Penguin, 1984.

Wolfe, Sidney, and Christopher Coley. *Pills That Don't Work*. Washington, DC: Public Citizen Press, 1980.

Retirement Housing

AARP. *Home-Made Money: Consumer's Guide to Home Equity Conversion*. Washington, DC: AARP Books, 1987.

Adelmann, Nora E. *Directory of Life Care Communities: A Guide to Retirement Communities for Independent Living*. New York: W. H. Wilson, 1981.

American Association of Homes for the Aging. *Continuing Care Homes: A Guidebook for Consumers*. Washington, DC: American Association of Homes for the Aging, 1990.

Bierbrier, Doreen. *Living with Tenants: How to Happily Share Your House with Renters for Profit and Security*. Arlington, Va.: The Housing Connection, 1983.

Boardman, John. *Living on Wheels: The Complete Guide to Motor Homes*. Summit, Pa.: Blue Ridge, 1987.

Burger, Sarah Greene. *Living in a Nursing Home: A Complete Guide for Residents*. New York: Continuum, 1988.

Bush, Vanessa. *Condominiums and Cooperatives: Everything You Need to Know*. Chicago: Contemporary Books, 1986.

Carlin, Vivian, and Ruth Mansberg. *If I Live to Be One Hundred: Congregate Housing for Later Life*. Englewood Cliffs, NJ: Prentice-Hall, 1984.

Cosby, Robert, and Terri Flynn. *Housing for Older Adults: Options and Answers*. Washington, DC: National Council on the Aging, 1986.

Gold, Margaret. *Guide to Housing Alternatives for Older Consumers*. Mount Vernon, NY: Consumer Reports Books, 1985.

Hare, Patrick. *Accessory Apartments: Using Surplus Space in Single-Family Houses*. Chicago: American Planning Association, 1981.

Harrison, Harry S., and Margery B. Leonard. *Homebuying: The Complete Illustrated Guide*. Chicago: National Association of Realtors, 1980.

Hemming, Roy, ed. *Finding the Right Place for Your Retirement*. New York: 50-Plus Guidebooks, 1983.

Horne, Jo, and Leo Baldwin. *Homesharing and Other Lifestyle Options*. Washington, DC: AARP Books, 1988.

Kennedy, David. *The Condominium and Cooperative Apartment Buyer's and Seller's Guide*. New York: Wiley, 1987.

Mongeau, Sam, ed. *Directory of Nursing Homes*. Phoenix: Oryx Press, 1988.

Myers, Phyllis. *Aging in Place: Strategies to Help the Elderly Stay in Revitalizing Neighborhoods*. Washington, DC: Conservation Foundation, 1982.

Osterbind, Carter, ed. *Independent Living for Older People*. Gainesville, Fla.: University Presses of Florida, 1972.

Raper, Ann T. *National Continuing Care Directory*. Des Plaines, Ill.: Scott, Foresman and Company, 1987.

Raschko, Bettyann. *Housing Interiors for the Disabled and Elderly*. New York: Van Nostrand, 1982.

Shared Housing Resource Center. *Shared Housing for Older People: A Planning Manual for Match-Up Programs*. Philadelphia: National Shared Housing Resource Center, 1983.

Wolfe, Laura. *Living in a Motor Home*. New Hope, Pa.: Woodsong Graphics, 1984.

Woodall's Retirement Directory. Highland Park, Ill.: Woodall Publishing Company, 1985.

Financial Matters

AARP. *Your Vital Papers Logbook*. Washington, DC: AARP Worker Equity Department, 1984.

Barnes, John. *More Money for Your Retirement*. New York: Harper & Row, 1978.

Chase, Nancy. *Policy-Wise: The Practical Guide to Insurance Decisions for Older Consumers*. Washington, DC: AARP Books, 1985.

Clay, William. *Guide to Estate Planning*. Homewood, Ill.: Dow Jones–Irwin, 1982.

Clifford, Denis. *Nolo's Simple Will Book*. Berkeley, Calif.: Nolo Press, 1986.

Donoghue, William. *Investment Tips for Retirement Savings*. New York: Harper & Row, 1987.

Dorfman, John. *Family Investment Guide*. New York: Jove Books, 1984.

Downes, John, and Jordan Goodman. *Dictionary of Finance and Investment Terms*. Hauppauge, NY: Barron's, 1985.

Hughes, Theodore, and David Klein. *Family Guide to Wills, Funerals, and Probate: How to Protect Yourself and Your Survivors*. New York: Scribner's, 1987.

Jehle, Faustin. *The Complete and Easy Guide to Social Security and Medicare*. Guilford, Conn.: Fraser, 1985.

Loewinsohn, Ruth. *Survival Handbook for Widows*. Des Plaines, Ill.: Scott, Foresman and Company, 1984.

Money Management Institute. *Money Management Library* (boxed set of booklets). Prospect Heights, Ill.: Household Financial Corporation, 1990.

North American Security Administrators Association (with the Council of Better Business Bureaus). *Investor Alert! How to Protect Your Money from Schemes, Scams, and Frauds*. Kansas City, MO: Andrews & McMeel, 1988.

Nuaheim, Fred. *The Retirement Money Book*. Washington, DC: Acropolis Books, 1982.

Plotnik, Charles, and Stephan Leimberg. *Keeping Your Money: How to Avoid Taxes and Probate through Estate Planning*. New York: Wiley, 1987.

Porter, Sylvia. *New Money Book for the 1990s*. New York: Avon, 1990.

Quinn, Jane B. *Everyone's Money Book*. New York: Delacorte Press, 1979.

Seskin, Jane. *Alone—Not Lonely: Independent Living for Women Over Fifty*. Washington, DC: AARP Books, 1985.

Sloan, Leonard. *The New York Times Book of Personal Finance*. New York: Times Books, 1990.

Soled, Alex J. *The Essential Guide to Wills, Estates, Trusts, and Death Taxes*. Des Plaines, Ill.: Scott, Foresman and Company, 1984.

Sutkowski, Edward. *Estate Planning: A Basic Guide*. Chicago: American Bar Association, 1986.

Train, John. *Preserving Capital and Making It Grow*. New York: Penguin Books, 1983.

Weaver, Peter, and Annette Buchanan. *What to Do with What You've Got*. Washington, DC: AARP Books, 1986.

Weinstein, Grace. *The Lifetime Book of Money Management*. New York: New American Library, 1985.

Legal Matters

AARP. *Legal Rights Calendar*. Washington, DC: AARP Books, 1991.

Alderman, Richard. *Know Your Rights!* Houston: Gulf Publishing Company, 1986.

Belli, Melvin, and Allen Wilkinson. *Everybody's Guide to the Law*. New York: Harper & Row, 1987.

Campbell, Roger, ed. *The Better Business Bureau A to Z Buying Guide*. New York: Henry Holt, 1990.

Jacoby and Meyers. *Practical Guide to Everyday Law*. New York: Simon & Schuster, 1986.

Legal Counsel for the Elderly. *Elderly Law Manual*. Washington, DC: AARP Books, 1990.

MacFarlane, G. *Layman's Dictionary of Law*. Elmsford, NJ: Pergamon Books, 1984.

Random House Editors. *You and the Law*. New York: Random House, 1988.

Persico, J. E., and George Sunderland. *Keeping Out of Crime's Way*. Des Plaines, Ill.: Scott, Foresman and Company, 1988.

Reader's Digest Editors. *Consumer Advisor: An Action Guide to Your Rights*. Pleasantville, NY: Reader's Digest Association, 1984.

Smith, Wesley. *The Lawyer Book: Everything You Always Wanted to Know about Lawyers but Didn't Have the Nerve to Ask*. Los Angeles: Price/Stern/Sloan, 1986.

Wishard, William. *Rights of the Elderly and Retired: A People's Handbook*. Oakland, Calif.: Cragmont, 1979.

Yates, Sharon F., ed. *Legal Question & Answer Book*. Pleasantville, NY: Reader's Digest Association, 1988.

Death and Bereavement

Caine, Lynn. *Widow*. New York: Bantam Books, 1975.

Consumer Reports Editors. *Funerals: Consumers' Last Rights*. New York: Pantheon Books, 1979.

Duda, Deborah. *Coming Home: A Guide to Health Care for the Terminally Ill*. Santa Fe, NM: Muir, 1984.

Gatov, Elisabeth. *Widows in the Dark*. New York: Warner Books, 1986.

Kubler-Ross, Elisabeth. *Living with Death and Dying*. New York: Macmillan, 1981.

Lewis, Albert, and Florence Kulick. *Survival Manual for Widows and Widowers*. East Hampton, NY: Carriage House, 1988.

Nelson, T. C. *It's Your Choice: The Practical Guide to Planning a Funeral*. Washington, DC: AARP Books, 1982.

O'Connor, Nancy. *Letting Go with Love: The Grieving Process*. Apache Junction, Ariz.: La Mariposa Press, 1985.

Parkes, C. M., and R. Weiss. *Recovery from Bereavement*. New York: Basic Books, 1983.

Schoen, Elin, and Pat Gobitz. *Widower*. New York: William Morrow and Company, 1984.

Stearns, Ann K. *Living through Personal Crisis*. New York: Ballantine Books, 1984.

Travel, Sports, and Recreation for Older People

Barish, Frances. *Frommer's Guide for the Disabled Traveler*. Englewood Cliffs, NJ: Prentice-Hall, 1984.

Carlson, Raymond, ed. *National Directory of Budget Motels*. Babylon, NY: Pilot Books, 1988.

Cohen, Marjorie. *Volunteer! The Comprehensive Guide to Voluntary Service*. Yarmouth, Me.: Intercultural Press, 1984.

DeVries, Herbert, and Dianne Hales. *Fitness Over Fifty: An Exercise Prescription for Lifelong Health*. New York: Scribner's, 1987.

Grimes, Paul. *The New York Times Practical Traveler*. New York: Times Books, 1985.

Hawkins, Gary. *USA by Bus and Train*. New York: Pantheon, 1985.

Hecker, Helen. *Directory of Travel Agencies for the Disabled*. Vancouver, Wash.: Twin Peaks Press, 1988.

Heilman, Joan. *Unbelievably Good Deals and Great Adventures You Absolutely Can't Get Unless You're Over 50*. Pullman, Wash.: Golden Companions Books, 1989.

LaBuda, Dennis. *The Gadget Book*. Des Plaines, Ill.: Scott, Foresman and Company, 1985.

Ley, Olga. *Exercises for Non-Athletes Over Fifty-one*. New York: Schocken Books, 1987.

Martin, Robert. *Fly There for Less: Seventy Ways to Save Money Flying Worldwide*. Teakwood Press, 1989.

Massow, Rosalind. *Travel Easy: The Practical Guide for People Over 50*. Des Plaines, Ill.: Scott, Foresman and Company, 1985.

McMillon, Bill. *Volunteer Vacations*. Chicago: Chicago Review Press, 1987.

National Park Foundation. *The Complete Guide to America's National Parks*. New York: Penguin Books, 1988.

Palmer, Paige. *Senior Citizen's Guide to Budget Travel in Europe*. Babylon, NY: Pilot Books, 1988.

Ralston, Jeannie. *Walking for the Health of It*. Washington, DC: AARP Books, 1987.

Rundbak, Betty, and Nancy Kramer. *Bed and Breakfast, USA*. New York: Dutton, 1988.

Simmons, Richard. *Reach for Fitness: A Special Book of Exercises for the Physically Challenged*. New York: Warner, 1986.

Sloan, Steven. *The Pocket Guide to Safe Travel*. Chicago: Contemporary Books, 1988.

Springer, Marilyn, and Don Schultz. *Dollarwise Guide to Cruises from the United States*. Englewood Cliffs, NJ: Prentice-Hall, 1984.

Warren, Stuart. *Bus Touring: A Guide to Charter Vacations*. Santa Fe, NM: Muir, 1988.

Webster, Harriet. *Trips for Those Over Fifty*. Portsmouth, NH: Yankee Books, 1988.

Weintz, Carol, and Walter Weintz. *The Discount Guide for Travelers Over 55*. New York: Dutton, 1988.

Wright, Don. *Guide to Free Campgrounds*. Charlotte, Vt.: Williamson Publishing Company, 1987.

INDEX

321